Manual for Eye Examination and Diagnosis

Mark W. Leitman MD

Attending Physician
Robert Wood Johnson Hospital and St Peter's Medical Center.
New Brunswick, New Jersey

FOURTH EDITION

BOSTON
Blackwell Scientific Publications
OXFORD LONDON EDINBURGH
MELBOURNE PARIS BERLIN VIENNA

© 1994 by
Blackwell Scientific Publications, Inc.
Editorial offices:
238 Main Street, Cambridge
  Massachusetts 02142, USA
Osney Mead, Oxford OX2 0EL, England
25 John Street, London WC1N 2BL
  England
23 Ainslie Place, Edinburgh EH3 6AJ
  Scotland
54 University Street, Carlton
  Victoria 3053, Australia

Other editorial offices:
Librairie Arnette SA
1, rue de Lille
75007 Paris
France

Blackwell Wissenschafts-Verlag GmbH
Düsseldorfer Str. 38
D-10707 Berlin
Germany

Blackwell MZV
Feldgasse 13
A-1238 Wien
Austria

First published 1975
Fourth edition 1994

Set by Setrite Typesetters Ltd, Hong Kong
Printed and bound in Hong Kong by
Dah Hua Printing Press Co. Ltd

94 95 96 97 5 4 3 2 1

DISTRIBUTORS

USA
  Blackwell Scientific Publications, Inc.
  238 Main Street
  Cambridge, Massachusetts 02142
  (*Orders*: Tel: 800 759−6102
              617 876−7000)

Canada
  Times Mirror
  Professional Publishing Ltd
  130 Flaska Drive
  Markham, Ontario L6G 1B8
  (*Orders*: Tel: 800 268−4178
              416 470−6739)

Australia
  Blackwell Scientific Publications Pty Ltd
  54 University Street
  Carlton, Victoria 3053
  (*Orders*: Tel: 03 347−5552)

  Outside North America and Australia
    Marston Book Services Ltd
    PO Box 87
    Oxford OX2 0DT
    (*Orders*: Tel: 0865 791155
                Fax: 0865 791927
                Telex: 837515)

Library of Congress
Cataloging-in-Publication Data

Leitman, Mark W., 1946−
    Manual for eye examination and
    diagnosis/Mark W. Leitman. 4th ed.
        p.   cm.
    Rev. ed. of: Manual for eye examination
    and diagnosis. 3rd ed. c1988.
    ISBN 0−86542−339−3
    1. Eye−Examination−Handbooks,
    manuals, etc. 2. Eye−Diseases and
    defects−Diagnosis−Handbooks,
    manuals, etc. I. Leitman, Mark W.,
    1946−   Manual for eye examination
    and diagnosis. II. Title.
    [DNLM: 1. Eye Diseases−diagnosis−
    handbooks.
    WW 39 L533m 1994]
    RE75.L44   1994
    617.7′15−dc20

Contents

Preface

This manual was written to help prevent students from being overwhelmed when performing their first eye examination. Since few students have the time to read and absorb hundreds of pages of introductory text prior to their first exposure to examining patients' eyes, each sentence in this manual was carefully chosen to present basic vocabulary and concepts vital to the practice of ophthalmology.

The material is presented in the order of an eye examination. Clinical findings at each step of the examination are discussed with respect to anatomy, differential diagnosis, instruments, and treatment. The book is designed to impart a basic understanding of how an ophthalmologist spends 95% of his or her day.

My appreciation goes to two former teachers, Dr Paul Henkind and Dr Sam Gartner, who assisted me in preparing the first two editions. When the publisher told me I could add the 211 color photos to this edition, I turned to an old friend, Joseph Walsh, chairman of the New York Eye and Ear Infirmary. His outstanding medical photographer, Denise Hess, contributed most of the unlabeled photos.

The broad acceptance of the previous editions over the past 18 years mandated this fourth, updated edition and translations into Japanese, Italian, Spanish, and Indonesian.

The additional color photos should further enhance your perspective of this fascinating specialty. I hope you enjoy it and appreciate it as an overview and supplement it with appropriate references.

MARK W. LEITMAN

Medical history

The history includes the patient's chief complaints, medical illnesses, current medications, allergies to medications, and family history of eye disease.

Common chief complaints	Causes
Persistent loss of vision	1 Focusing problems are the most common complaints. Everyone eventually needs glasses to attain perfect vision, and fitting lenses occupies half the ophthalmologist's day 2 Cataracts are cloudy lenses that reduce vision in half the people over 70 years of age. Unoperated cataracts are the leading cause of blindness worldwide. In the USA, over 1.3 million cataract extractions are performed each year 3 Diabetes affects 14 million Americans, increasing from 0.3% at age 20 to 10% of the population after age 70. Diabetic retinopathy is the leading cause of blindness in the USA in those under 65 years of age 4 Macular degeneration causes loss of central vision and is the leading cause of blindness over age 65. Signs are present in 25% of people over age 75 5 Glaucoma is elevated eye pressure that damages the optic nerve. It usually occurs after age 35 and affects 2 million Americans with black persons affected five times as often as white persons. Peripheral vision is lost first, with no symptoms until it is far advanced. Progression to blindness is uncommon if discovered early. This is why there are so many state-sponsored eye-pressure screenings
Transient loss of vision lasting less than $\frac{1}{2}$ hour, with or without flashing lights	In persons over age 45, microemboli from arteriosclerotic plaques cause transient blurring as they pass through the eye or visual cortex, whereas in younger individuals it is often a migrainous spasm of an artery causing these symptoms
Floaters	Almost everyone will at some time see shifting spots due to suspended particles in the normally clear vitreous. They are usually physiologic, but may result from hemorrhage, retinal detachments, or other serious conditions
Flashes of light	Sparks may be due to traction of the vitreous on the retina and are sometimes associated with the onset of a retinal hole or detachment. Insults to the visual

Continued on p. 2

Common chief complaints (Cont.)	Causes (Cont.)
	center in the occipital cortex are usually ischemic and cause more organized jagged lines of light
Night blindness (nyctalopia)	Nyctalopia usually indicates a need for spectacle change, but also commonly occurs with aging and cataracts. Rarer causes include retinitis pigmentosa and vitamin A deficiency
Double vision (diplopia)	Strabismus, which affects 4% of the population, is the condition where the eyes are not looking in the same direction. The binocular diplopia disappears when one eye is covered. In straight-eyed persons, diplopia is caused by hysteria or a beam-splitting opacity in one eye which does not disappear by covering the other eye
Light sensitivity (photophobia)	Usually a normal condition treated with tinted lenses, but could result from inflammation of the eye or brain; internal reflection of light in lightly pigmented or albinotic eyes; or dispersion of light by mucus, lens or corneal opacities, or retinal degeneration
Itching	Most often due to allergy or dry eye, which affects 30% of elderly persons
Headache	Headache patients present daily to rule out eye causes and to seek direction. 1 Headache due to blurred vision or eye-muscle imbalance worsens with use of eyes 2 Tension causes 80–90% of headaches. It worsens with anxiety and is often associated with temple and neck pain 3 Migraine occurs in 10% of the population. There is a severe recurrent, pounding headache often accompanied by nausea, blurred vision, and flashing zigzag lights. It is relieved by rest 4 Sinusitis causes a dull ache about the eyes and occasional tenderness over the sinus. There may be an associated nasal stuffiness and a history of allergy relieved with decongestants 5 Menstrual headaches are cyclical 6 Giant-cell arteritis occurs in elderly persons and may cause headache, loss of vision, pain on chewing, temporal scalp tenderness, arthritis, loss of weight, and weakness. An erythrocyte sedimentation rate over 40 and a positive temporal artery biopsy confirms the diagnosis. Prompt high-dose systemic steroid therapy should be started since blindness or death can occur 7 Sharp ocular pains lasting for seconds are often referred from nerve irritations in the neck, nasal mucosa, or intracranial dura, which are also innervated by the trigeminal nerve 8 Headaches that awaken the patient and are prolonged, or associated with focal neurologic symptoms should referred for neurologic study

Medical illnesses

Record all systemic diseases. Ophthalmologists commonly see patients with diabetes mellitus and thyroid disease. Both are often first discovered in an eye examination.

Diabetes mellitus

1 Diabetes may be first diagnosed when there are large changes in spectacle correction due to the effect of blood sugar changes on the lens of the eye.

2 Diabetes is one of the common causes of III, IV, and VI cranial nerve paralysis, which is due to closure of small vessels. The resulting diplopia may be the first symptom of diabetes.

3 Cataracts are more common and occur at a younger age in diabetics.

4 Retinopathy is the most serious complication. It rarely occurs at the onset of the disease, but is present in 25% of eyes by 10 years and 80% by 20 years of age. Once it appears, the patient should be examined yearly or more often, since laser treatment reduces visual complications by 50%.

Autoimmune (Graves') thyroid disease

This is a condition in which an orbitopathy may be present with hyper- but also hypo- or euthyroid disease.

1 It is the most common cause of bulging eyes referred to as exophthalmos or proptosis, and is due to white-cell and mucopolysaccharide infiltration of the orbit. A small white area of sclera appearing between the lid and upper cornea is diagnostic of thyroid disease 90% of the time (Fig. 1). This exposed sclera may be a result of exophthalmos or thyroid lid retraction due to an overactive Muller's muscle that elevates the lid. Severe orbitopathy may be treated with steroids, radiation, or surgical decompression of the orbit.

2 Infiltration of eye muscles may cause diplopia and is confirmed by a computed tomography (CT) scan (Fig. 2) or magnetic resonance imaging (MRI).

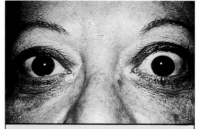

Fig. 1 Thyroid exophthalmos with exposed sclera at superior limbus.

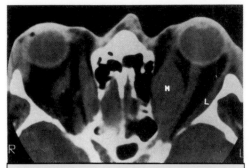

Fig. 2 Computed tomography scan of thyroid orbitopathy showing infiltration of medial rectus muscle (M) and normal lateral rectus muscle (L). Courtesy of Jack Rootman.

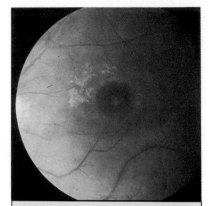

Fig. 3 Bull's eye maculopathy due to Plaquenil.

3 Exophthalmos may cause excessive exposure of the eye in the day and an inability to close the lids at night (lagophthalmos), resulting in damage to the cornea.

4 Optic nerve compression could cause permanent loss of vision.

Medications

Record patient medications. Below are listed the most commonly prescribed drugs causing side effects that necessitate routine eye examinations.

Plaquenil used for autoimmune diseases and malaria causes "bulls-eye" maculopathy (Fig. 3).

Ethambutol used for tuberculosis causes optic neuritis.

Phenothiazine tranquilizers cause macular degeneration (Fig. 4).

Corticosteroids cause cataracts (Fig. 5), glaucoma, and herpes keratitis.

Mevocor, used to lower cholesterol, causes cataracts.

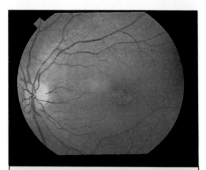

Fig. 4 Phenothiazine maculopathy.

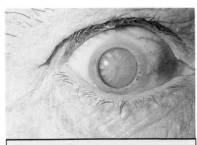

Fig. 5 Cataract.

Allergies to medications

Inquire about drug allergies before eye drops are placed or medications prescribed. Neomycin, a popular antibiotic in eye drops, may cause conjunctivitis and reddened skin (Fig. 6).

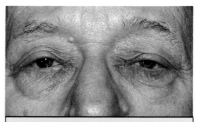

Fig. 6 Neomycin allergy occurs in 5–10% of population.

Family history of eye disease

Cataracts, refractive errors, retinal degeneration, and strabismus — to name a few — may all be inherited. In glaucoma, which normally affects 1% of the population, family members have a 10% chance of acquiring the disease. Eighty percent of people with migraine have a relative with the disease.

Measurement of vision and refraction

Visual acuity

The patients read the Snellen chart (Fig. 7) from 20 ft with the left eye occluded first. Take the vision in each eye without and then with spectacles.

Vision is expressed in a fraction-like form. The top number is the distance at which the patient reads the chart; the bottom number is the distance at which someone with normal vision reads the same line of the chart. Whenever acuity is less than 20/20, determine the cause for the decreased vision. The most common cause is a refractive error, i.e., the need for lens correction.

If visual acuity is less than 20/20, the patient may be examined with a pinhole. Improvement of vision while looking through a pinhole indicates that spectacles will improve vision. Use an illiterate "E" chart with a young child or an illiterate adult.

Ask the patient which way the ∃ is pointed. Near vision is checked with a reading card held about 14 inches away. If a refraction for new spectacles is necessary, perform it prior to other tests that may disturb the eye.

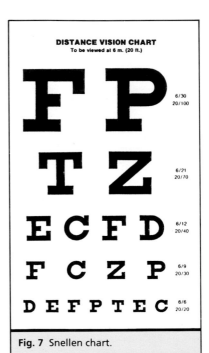

DISTANCE VISION CHART
To be viewed at 6 m. (20 ft.)

F P	6/30 20/100
T Z	6/21 20/70
E C F D	6/12 20/40
F C Z P	6/9 20/30
D E F P T E C	6/6 20/20

Fig. 7 Snellen chart.

Examples of visual acuity

Measurement in feet (meters in parentheses)	Meaning
20/20 (6/6)	Normal. At 20 ft, patient reads a line that a normal eye sees at 20 ft
20/30−2 (6/9−2)	Missed two letters of 20/30 line
20/50 (6/15)	Vision required in at least one eye for driver's license in most states

Continued

Measurement in feet (meters in parentheses)	Meaning
20/200 (6/60)	Legally blind. At 20 ft, patient reads line that normal eye could see at 200 ft
10/400 (3/120)	If patient cannot read top line at 20 ft, walk him or her to the chart. Record as the "numerator" the distance at which the top line first becomes clear
CF/2 ft (counts fingers at 2 ft)	If patient is unable to read top line at 3 ft, have the patient count fingers at maximal distance
HM/3 ft (hand motion at 3 ft)	If at 1 ft patient cannot count fingers, ask him or her direction of hand motion
LP/Proj. (light perception with projection)	Light perception with ability to determine position of the light
NLP	No light perception: totally blind

Record vision as follows			Key	
\s̄/ V	OD	20/70+1	V	Vision
	OS	LP/Proj.	s̄	Without spectacles
			c̄	With spectacles
			OD	Right eye
\c̄/ V	OD	20/20	OS	Left eye
	OS	LP/Proj.	OU	Both eyes

Optics

Emmetropia (no refractive error)

In an emmetropic eye (Fig. 8), light from a distance is focused on the retina.

Ametropia

In this disorder, light is not focused on the retina. Four types are hyperopia, myopia, astigmatism, and presbyopia.

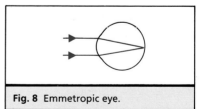

Fig. 8 Emmetropic eye.

Hyperopia

Parallel rays of light are focused behind the retina (Fig. 9). The patient is farsighted and sees more clearly at a distance than near, but still might require glasses for distance.

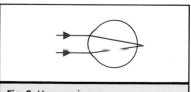

Fig. 9 Hyperopic eye.

A convex positive lens is used to correct hyperopia (Fig. 10). The power of the lens is expressed in diopters (D), which range from +0.25 to +20.00. A positive 1 D lens converges parallel rays of lights to a focus 1 meter from the lens (Fig. 11). The total refracting power of the eye is 60 D; 43 D from the cornea and 17 D from the lens.

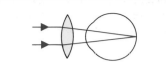

Fig. 10 Hyperopic eye corrected with convex lens.

Myopia

Parallel rays are focused in front of the retina (Fig. 12). The patient is nearsighted and sees more clearly near than at distance. Myopia often begins in the first decade and progresses until stabilization at the end of the second or third decade. One in four Americans are myopic.

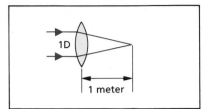

Fig. 11 Parallel rays focused by 1 D lens.

A concave negative lens (Fig. 13), which diverges light rays, is used to correct this condition.

Corrections range from −0.25 to −20.00 D.

Refractive myopia is due to increased curvature of the cornea or the human lens, whereas axial myopia is due to elongation of the eye. In axial myopia the retina is sometimes stretched so much that it pulls away from the optic disk (see Fig. 225, p. 77) and may cause retinal thinning (see Fig. 226, p. 77) with subsequent holes or detachments.

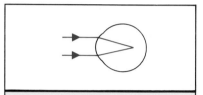

Fig. 12 Myopic eye.

Astigmatism

In this condition, which effects 85% of people, the rays entering the eye are not refracted uniformly in all meridians. Regular astigmatism occurs when the corneal curvature is uniformly different in meridians at right angles to each other. It is corrected with spectacles. For example, take the case of astigmatism in the horizontal (180°) meridian (Fig. 14). A slit beam of vertical light (AB) is focused on the retina, and (CD) anterior to the retina. To correct this regular astigmatism, a myopic cylindrical lens (Fig. 15) is used that diverges only CD.

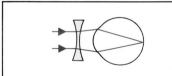

Fig. 13 Myopic eye corrected by concave lens.

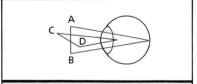

Fig. 14 Myopic astigmatism.

Irregular astigmatism is caused by a distorted cornea, usually resulting from an injury or a disease called keratoconus (see Fig. 125, p. 50).

Presbyopia

This is a decrease in near vision, which occurs in all people at about age 43. The normal eye has to adjust +2.50 D to change focus from distance to near. This is called accommodation. The eye's ability to accommodate decreases from +14 D at age 14 to +2 D at age 50.

Middle-aged persons are given reading glasses with plus lenses that require updating with age.

40–45 years	+1.00 to +1.50 D
50 years	+1.50 to +2.00 D
over 55 years	+2.00 to +2.50 D

The additional plus lens in a full reading glass (Fig. 16) blurs distance vision. Half glasses (Fig. 17) and bifocals (Fig. 18) are options that allow for clear distance vision when looking up. No-line bifocals are more attractive, but more expensive.

Refraction

Refraction is the technique of determining the lenses necessary to correct the optical defects of the eye.

Trial case and lenses

The lens case (Fig. 19) contains convex and concave spherical and cylindrical lenses and prisms. The diopter power of spherical lenses and the axis of cylindrical lenses are recorded on the lens frames.

Trial frame

The trial frame (Fig. 20) holds the trial lenses. Place the strongest spherical lenses in the compartment closest to the eye because the

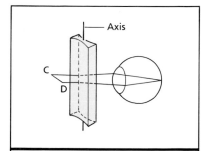

Fig. 15 Myopic astigmatism corrected with a myopic cylinder, axis 90°.

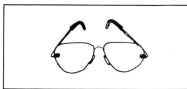

Fig. 16 Full reading glass blurs distance vision.

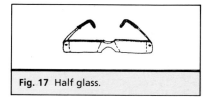

Fig. 17 Half glass.

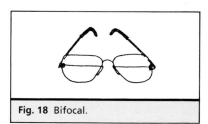

Fig. 18 Bifocal.

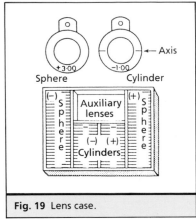

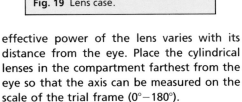

Fig. 19 Lens case.

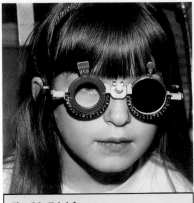

Fig. 20 Trial frame.

effective power of the lens varies with its distance from the eye. Place the cylindrical lenses in the compartment farthest from the eye so that the axis can be measured on the scale of the trial frame (0°−180°).

Streak retinoscopy ("flash")

This objective means of determining the refractive error is used to prescribe glasses to infants and illiterate persons who cannot give adequate subjective responses. Hold the retinoscope (Fig. 21) at arm's length from the eye and direct its linear beam onto the pupil. To determine the axis of astigmatism, rotate the beam until it parallels the pupillary reflex (Fig. 22), then move it back and forth at that axis, as demonstrated in Fig. 23.

If the reflex moves the same way that the retinoscope beam is moving ("with motion"),

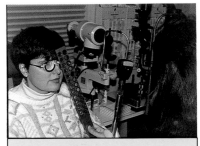

Fig. 21 Streak retinoscope.

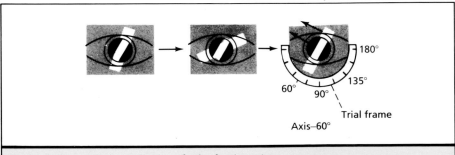

Fig. 22 Retinoscopic determination of axis of astigmatism.

a plus (+) lens is added to the trial frame. If the reflex moves in the opposite direction ("against motion"), a negative (−) lens is needed. Absence of "with motion" or "against motion" indicates the endpoint. Add −1.50 D to the above findings to approximate the refractive error of that meridian. Rotate the beam 90° to refract the other axis.

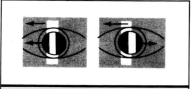

Fig. 23 Pupillary reflex with motion and against motion.

Manifest

A manifest is the subjective trial of lenses. Place the approximate lenses, as determined by the old spectacles or retinoscopy, in a trial frame. Occlude one of the patient's eyes, and refine the sphere by the addition of (+) and (−) 0.25 D lenses. Ask which lens makes the letters clearer. Next, refine the cylinder axis by rotating the lens in the direction of clearest vision. Test the cylinder power by adding (+) and (−) cylinders at that axis. Large changes in cylinder or axis may improve vision, but partial corrections are sometimes given to adults, since they find it difficult to adjust. Children are given the full cylinder.

In presbyopes, determine the reading "add" after distance correction.

The following abbreviations are used to record the results of the refraction: W, old spectacle prescription as determined in a lensometer; F, "flash", the refractive error by retinoscopy; M, manifest, the subjective correction by trial and error; Rx, final prescription, usually equal to M.

A bifocal prescription for a farsighted presbyope with astigmatism is written as follows:

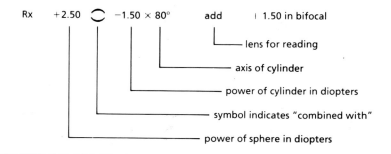

Plastic lenses are prescribed 90% of the time because they are lighter and have less chance of shattering, especially in children. Glass is heavier, but has the advantage of not scratching as easily. For photophobia, grey tints are often prescribed because they distort all colors equally.

Photochromic lenses darken in sunlight. Ultraviolet filters reduce the incidence of skin cancer, cataracts, and macular degeneration.

Contact lenses

Contacts are worn by 24 million Americans. Daily-wear soft lenses are the most common. They last about a year and are removed, cleaned, and sterilized each night. Disposable daily wear lenses that last for 2 weeks to 3 months are gaining in popularity because of a reduction in mucous deposits. Extended-wear lenses that remain in overnight for up to 2 weeks are more convenient, but have five times the risk of infection.

Hard and gas-permeable rigid lenses may correct astigmatism better, but are less comfortable. To fit contacts, a keratometer (Fig. 24) is used to measure the shape of the cornea. Lenses based on that curvature are then tried until sharp vision, good centering, and comfort are attained.

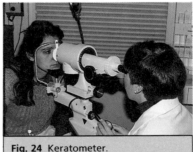

Fig. 24 Keratometer.

Radial keratotomy

This surgery has been used for over 10 years to correct refractive errors. To correct myopia, the cornea is flattened by making 4–8 radial incisions through 90% of the corneal depth. Problems such as inability to predict amount of correction, variable vision throughout the day, infection, cataract formation, glare, and corneal perforation (Fig. 25) have slowed widespread acceptance. Hopefully, the new laser technique (photorefractive keratectomy) will minimize some of these problems.

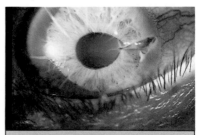

Fig. 25 Rare instance of traumatic rupture of radial keratotomy wound. Courtesy of Leo Bores.

Neuro-ophthalmology

Eye movements

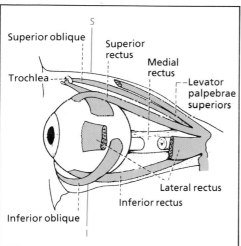

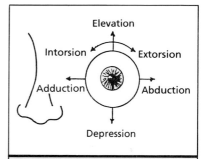

Fig. 27 The eye rotates around three different axes coordinated by the action of six extraocular muscles.

Fig. 26 Lateral orbital view: adduction and abduction is around vertical axis (S–I).

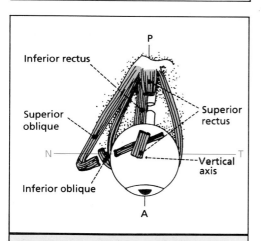

Fig. 28 Superior orbital view. Elevation and depression is on the horizontal axis (N–T) passing from the nasal to temporal side of the eye. Torsion is on the A–P axis.

Muscle	Actions	Neural control
Medial rectus	Adducts	Oculomotor nerve (CN III)
Inferior rectus	Mainly depresses, also extorts, adducts	Oculomotor nerve (CN III)
Superior rectus	Mainly elevates, also intorts, adducts	Oculomotor nerve (CN III)
Inferior oblique	Mainly extorts, also elevates, abducts	Oculomotor nerve (CN III)
Superior oblique	Mainly intorts, also depresses, abducts	Trochlear nerve (CN IV)
Lateral rectus	Abducts	Abducens nerve (CN VI)

CN, cranial nerve.

Strabismus

Strabismus refers to the nonalignment of the eyes such that an object in space is not visualized simultaneously by the fovea of each eye. Phoria refers to the potential for an eye to turn. Once it turns it is called a tropia.

Phoria

If one eye is occluded while both eyes are fusing, the occluded eye may turn in (esophoria, noted with the letter E) or out (exophoria, X). Small phorias are usually asymptomatic. Phorias degenerate into tropias as the amount of turn increases, and the patient's ability to correct it decreases. This

Types of tropias	
Esotropia (ET)	Deviation of eye nasally
Exotropia (XT)	Deviation of eye outward
Hypertropia (HT)	Deviation of eye upward
Intermittent tropia	A phoria that spontaneously breaks to a tropia; indicate with parentheses. Example R (ET) = right intermittent esotropia
Constant monocular tropia	Present at all times in one eye. Example: RXT, constant right exotropia. Often associated with loss of vision, if onset in childhood
Alternating tropia	Either eye can deviate. Vision is usually equal in both eyes

occurs with tiredness later in the day and from any stimulus that dissociates the eyes, such as poor vision in one eye. Absence of a phoria (perfectly straight eyes) is termed orthophoria.

Complications of strabismus

Amblyopia

Also called lazy eye, amblyopia is decreased vision due to improper use of an eye in childhood. The two common causes are an eyeturn (strabismic amblyopia) or a refractive error (refractive amblyopia), uncorrected before age 8. In strabismus, children unconsciously suppress the deviated eye to avoid diplopia. Strabismic amblyopia is treated by patching the good eye (Fig. 29), thereby forcing the child to use his amblyopic eye. Refractive amblyopia is treated by correcting the refractive error with glasses and patching the better eye. Both types must be treated in early childhood because after age 5, it is difficult to improve vision, and after age 8, it is almost impossible.

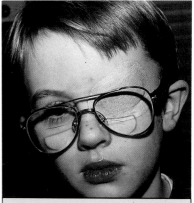

Fig. 29 Patching for amblyopia.

Poor cosmetic appearance

Tropias greater than 20 D that cannot be corrected with spectacles are often cosmetically unacceptable and require surgery.

Loss of fusion

Fusion occurs when the images from both eyes are perceived as one object, with resulting stereopsis (three-dimensional vision). Many patients with tropias never gain the ability to fuse. Finer grades of fusion are assessed by using the Wirt stereopsis test.

Wirt stereopsis test (Fig. 30)

While wearing polarized glasses, the patient views a special test card. The degree of fusion is determined by the number of pictures correctly described in three dimensions.

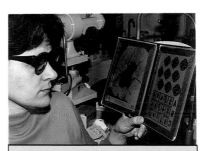

Fig. 30 Wirt stereopsis.

Near point of convergence (NPC) (Fig. 31)

The NPC is the closest point at which the eyes can cross to view a near object. It is measured by having the patient make a maximal effort to fixate on a small object as it is moved toward his or her eyes. The distance at which the eyes stop converging and one turns out is recorded as the NPC. Convergence insufficiency must be considered if the NPC is greater than 8 cm. These patients may complain of diplopia or other difficulties while reading. Exercises or prism glasses may help.

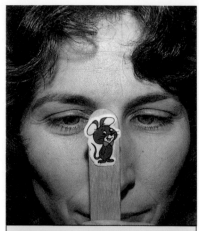

Fig. 31 Near point of convergence.

Accommodative esotropia
(Figs 32 and 33)

When the lens of a normal eye focuses, it simultaneously causes the eyes to converge. Hyperopes not wearing glasses must focus the lens of their eye (accommodation) to see clearly near and far. This focusing stimulates the accommodative reflex causing convergence of the eyes. When the ratio of convergence to accommodation is abnormally high an esotropia results, which corrects with lenses.

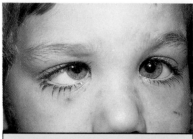

Fig. 32 Accommodative esotropia.

Nonaccommodative esotropia

This is due to a defect in the brain not related to the accommodative reflex. It is corrected by surgically weakening the medial rectus muscle by recessing its insertion posteriorly on the sclera (Fig. 34) or by tightening the lateral rectus muscle by resecting part of it (Fig. 35). Less often, botulinum toxin is injected to weaken eye muscles.

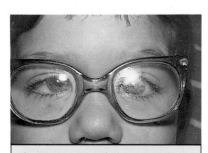

Fig. 33 Accommodative esotropia corrected with hyperopic lenses.

Measurement with prisms of the amount of eye-turn

Ocular deviations are measured in prism diopters. When light passes through a prism, it is bent toward the base of the prism. One

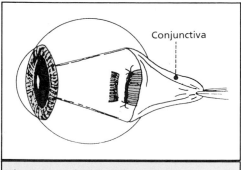

Fig. 34 Recession to weaken muscle.

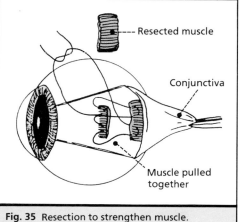

Fig. 35 Resection to strengthen muscle.

prism diopter (1 Δ) displaces the image 1 cm at a distance of 1 meter from the prism. Do not confuse prism diopters (Δ) with lens diopters (D).

In right esotropia, the right fovea is turned temporarily. To focus the light on the right fovea, a prism (apex-in) in placed in front of the right eye (Fig. 36). For an exotropia use apex-out. *Rule*: point prism apex in the direction of the tropia.

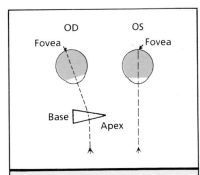

Fig. 36 Right esotropia neutralized with prism (apex-in).

Prism cover test for measurement of eye-turn (Fig. 37)

The patient fixates on an object at 20 ft. When the fixating eye is occluded, the deviated eye must move to look at the target. Increasing amounts of prism are placed in front of the deviated eye until no movement is noted when the cover is moved back and forth over each eye.

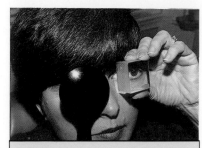

Fig. 37 Prism cover test.

Hirschberg's test

When the cover test is difficult to perform on young children, the angle of strabismus can be estimated by using Hirschberg's test (Figs 38–40). As the child fixates on a point source of light, the position of the corneal light reflexes are noted. Each 1 mm of deviation from the center of the cornea is equivalent to approximately 14 Δ of deviation. A reflex 2 mm temporal to the center of the cornea indicates an esotropia of approximately 28 Δ.

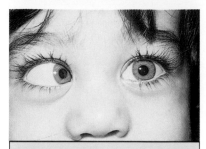

Fig. 38 Hirschberg: esotropia.

Causes of strabismus

1 Paralytic strabismus is due to cranial nerve (III, IV, or VI) disease or eye-muscle weakness from thyroid disease, traumatic contusions, myasthenia gravis, or orbital floor fractures.
2 Nonparalytic strabismus is due to a malfunction of a center in the brain. It is often inherited and begins in childhood.

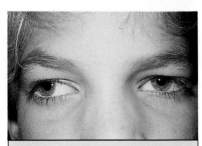

Fig. 39 Hirschberg: exotropia.

Demonstration of paralytic strabismus

In paralytic strabismus, the amount of deviation is greatest when gaze is directed in the field of action of the weakened muscle. To demonstrate underaction of any of the 12 external ocular muscles, the patient fixates an object moved into each of the six cardinal fields of gaze (Fig. 41). Each position tests one muscle of each eye (e.g., position 3 tests the right inferior rectus and the left superior

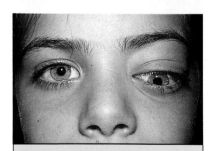

Fig. 40 Hirschberg: hypotropia.

Comparison of paralytic and nonparalytic strabismus

	Paralytic	Nonparalytic
Age of Onset	Usually in older persons	Usually starts before 6 years of age
Complaint	Diplopia	Cosmetic eyeturn; less diplopia since child suppresses deviated eye
Eye-turn	Largest deviation in field of action of affected muscle	No one muscle is underactive; deviation similar in all directions
Vision	Not affected	Deviated eye may have loss of vision (amblyopia)
Plan	Neurologic workup	Ophthalmic workup

oblique muscles). In addition to observing for underaction or overaction of the muscles, ask the patient where diplopia is greatest. For exact measurements, use the prism cover test.

Most often the cause for CN III, IV, and VI paralysis cannot be confirmed, since it is due to ischemia from small-vessel closure. Testing is done to rule out causes such as multiple sclerosis, aneurysms, neoplasms, and other rarer conditions, especially in younger individuals where vessel closure is not likely. Ischemia from diabetes is the most common cause and often resolves within 10 weeks.

CN III paralysis (Figs 42, 43, and 44) results in underaction of the inferior oblique and medial, inferior, and superior rectus muscles resulting in an eye turned down and out. Since this nerve also innervates the levator palpebral muscle, which elevates the lid and the pupillary constrictor muscle, the lid is drooped and the pupil is dilated (Fig. 42). CN

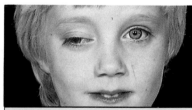

Fig. 42 Right CN III paralysis. In straight gaze, eye turns down and out with dilated pupil and ptosis.

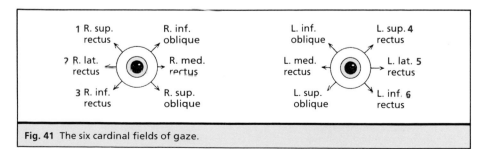

Fig. 41 The six cardinal fields of gaze.

In the left diagram (right eye):
- 1 R. sup. rectus
- R. inf. oblique
- 2 R. lat. rectus
- R. med. rectus
- 3 R. inf. rectus
- R. sup. oblique

In the right diagram (left eye):
- L. inf. oblique
- L. sup. 4 rectus
- L. med. rectus
- L. lat. 5 rectus
- L. sup. oblique
- L. inf. 6 rectus

III paralysis due to diabetes often spares the pupil.

Always examine for a dilated pupil after head trauma. CN III parallels the posterior communicating artery (Fig. 45, p. 21) so that ruptured aneurysms in the circle of Willis are a common cause of CN III paralysis with a dilated pupil and pain. Also, CN III passes under the tentorial ridge in the brain and is highly susceptible to uncal herniation of the brain. Herniation may follow increased intracranial pressure from cerebral edema, hematoma, tumor, abscess, or cerebral spinal fluid obstruction. Although a dilated pupil is a more common ominous sign after head injury, small or unequal pupils could indicate serious insults to other parts of the brain.

The trochlear nerve (CN IV) innervates the superior oblique muscle. Since this muscle acts as a depressor when the eye is rotated nasally, patients have vertical diplopia when looking down to read. Since intorsion is this muscle's main action, there is a head tilt to the opposite shoulder so that the eye doesn't have to be intorted (Fig. 46). If the doctor forces the patient's head straight (Fig. 47), the superior rectus must act as an intorter. Since the superior rectus also elevates the eye as it intorts, vertical diplopia occurs (Fig. 47). A common cause of superior oblique muscle dysfunction is trauma since it passes through the trochlea (see Fig. 26, p. 13), where it is accessible to injury due to its location just under the superior nasal orbital rim.

The abducens nerve (CN VI) innervates the lateral rectus muscle that abducts the eye. The patient complains of diplopia and a cross-

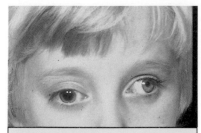

Fig. 43 Inability of right eye to look to the left due to medial rectus paralysis.

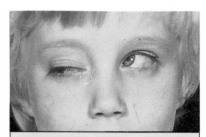

Fig. 44 Inability of right eye to look up to right due to superior rectus paralysis. Courtesy of David Taylor.

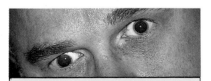

Fig. 46 Left superior oblique paralysis. To avoid diplopia, head is tilted to the opposite shoulder. Courtesy of Joseph Calhoun.

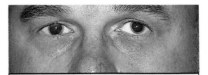

Fig. 47 Paralytic left superior oblique with vertical diplopia in primary gaze. Note: sclera visible below left cornea.

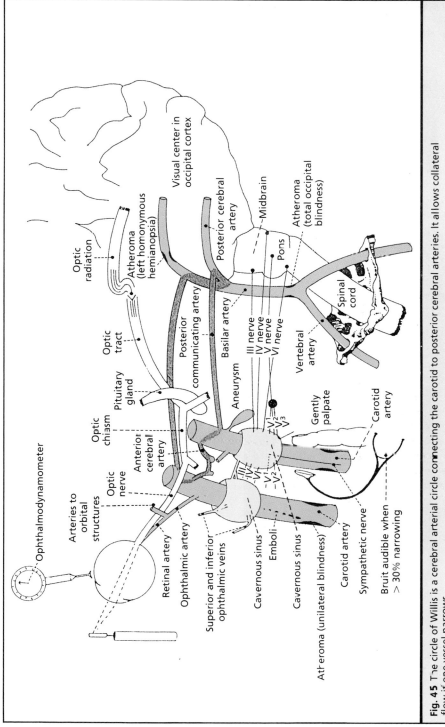

Fig. 45 The circle of Willis is a cerebral arterial circle connecting the carotid to posterior cerebral arteries. It allows collateral flow if one vessel narrows.

Ophthalmodynamometer

Arteries to orbital structures

Optic nerve

Retinal artery

Ophthalmic artery

Superior and inferior ophthalmic veins

Cavernous sinus

Emboli

Cavernous sinus

Atheroma (unilateral blindness)

Carotid artery

Sympathetic nerve

Bruit audible when > 30% narrowing

Carotid artery

Gently palpate

Vertebral artery

Spinal cord

Atheroma (total occipital blindness)

Pons

Midbrain

III nerve
IV nerve
V nerve
VI nerve

Aneurysm

Basilar artery

Posterior communicating artery

Posterior cerebral artery

Visual center in occipital cortex

Atheroma (left homonymous hemianopsia)

Optic radiation

Optic tract

Pituitary gland

Optic chiasm

Anterior cerebral artery

Optic nerve

eye (Figs 48–50). As this nerve may be damaged from increased intracranial pressure, one should be alert to an associated headache, nausea, and papilledema.

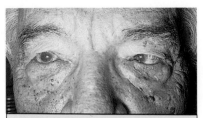

Fig. 48 Right lateral rectus paralysis in right gaze. Courtesy of Elliot Davidoff.

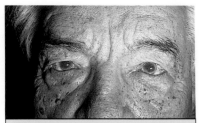

Fig. 49 Right lateral rectus paralysis straight gaze.

The trigeminal nerve (CN V) is the sensory nerve of the head and face (Fig. 51).

V^1: ophthalmic branch — sensory upper lid eye and nose.

V^2: maxillary branch — sensory to lower lid and cheek.

V^3: mandibular branch — no ocular action.

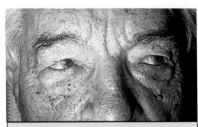

Fig. 50 Right lateral rectus paralysis left gaze.

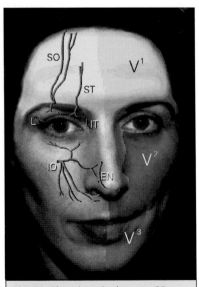

Fig. 51 The trigeminal nerve. SO, superior ophthalmic; ST, supratrochlear; L, lacrimal; IT, infratrochlear; IO, inferior ophthalmic; EN, external nasal.

Injury may cause an anesthetic effect, as occurs in an orbital blow-out fracture, or pain, as occurs in herpes zoster dermatitis (Fig. 52) or trigeminal neuralgia (tic douloureux).

Herpes zoster dermatitis (shingles) is caused by the virus also responsible for chicken pox. It often affects the ophthalmic division of CN V. There may be an associated iritis and keratitis when the side of the nose is involved since the nasociliary branch of CN V[1] supplies the eye and skin of the nose. There is usually a fever and adenopathy. Rx: acyclovir (Zovirax) 800 mg p.o. 5 times a day for dermatitis. The treatment for iritis is similar to other causes of iritis.

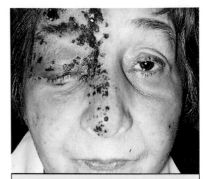

Fig. 52 Herpes zoster dermatitis.

The facial nerve (CN VII) innervates the orbicularis oculi muscle, which closes the lid, and also the muscles that control facial expression (Fig. 53). It also stimulates lacrimal secretion. The common paralysis in adults, Bell's palsy, is usually due to ischemia or a virus (Fig. 54).

The optic nerve (CN II) is made up of 1.2 million retinal ganglion cell axons (Figs 55 and 56). They transmit the visual message from the rods and cones of the eye to the brain (Fig. 56). The nerve begins at the optic disk (papilla) as the ganglion cell axons exit the eye. When the nerve is damaged, the normal orange disk turns chalk white (optic atrophy) (Figs 57 and 58). This may follow an intraocular insult to the retinal nerve fibers, as occurs with retinal artery occlusion or high intraocular pressure, (Fig. 59) or it may be caused by an extraocular insult to the nerve (optic neuropathy).

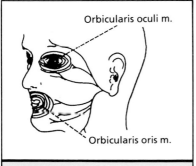

Orbicularis oculi m.

Orbicularis oris m.

Fig.53 Facial nerve to orbicularis oculi and oris muscles.

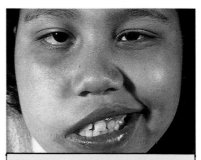

Fig. 54 Right CN VII paralysis causes decreased blinking and inability to close lids completely (Fig. 137).

Optic neuropathy involving the anterior nerve may cause swelling of the optic disk (papillitis) (Fig. 60). In papillitis there are sometimes flame hemorrhages around the disk, cells in the overlying vitreous, and a blurred disk margin. Optic neuropathy causes reduced central vision, decreased pupil reaction to light, reduced color vision, and pain with eye movement. Fifty percent of cases are due to multiple sclerosis. The next most common cause is ischemic optic neuropathy due to arteriosclerosis, diabetes, or giant cell arteritis. Less common etiologies are drug or tobacco–alcohol toxicity, folic acid or vitamin B_{12} deficiency,

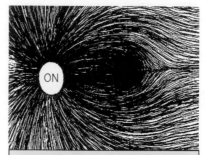

Fig. 55 Drawing of retinal nerve fiber layer with 1.2 million ganglion cell axons converging to make up the optic nerve (ON).

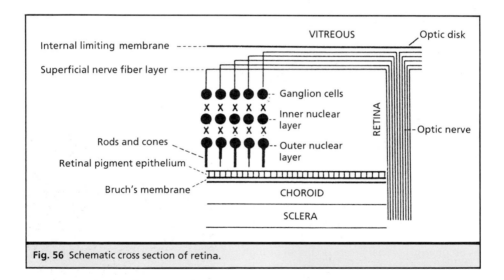

Fig. 56 Schematic cross section of retina.

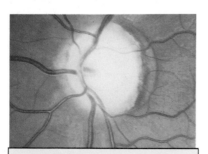

Fig. 57 Optic atrophy resulting from ischemia, transection, toxicity, or inflammation.

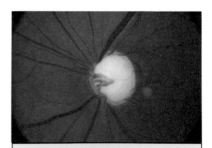

Fig. 58 Optic atrophy with cupping due to glaucoma.

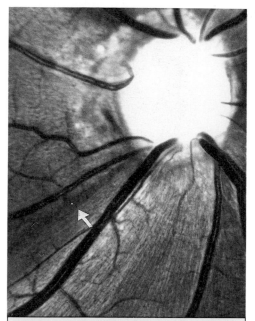

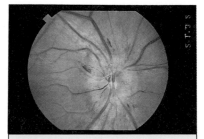

Fig. 60 Optic neuropathy with papillitis.

Fig. 59 "Red-free" photograph of glaucomatous cupping and loss of retinal nerve fiber layer (white arrows). The dark area with loss of striations is pathognomic of fiber loss if it fans out and widens further from disk. Courtesy of Michael P. Kelly.

trauma, compression from orbital inflammations, tumors, or thyroid disease, and a host of rarer inherited or neurologic diseases.

Multiple sclerosis is a chronic relapsing condition with a usual onset between the third and fifth decades. It is due to multiple areas of demyelination in the central nervous system (Fig. 61). Diplopia due to CN III, IV, or VI paralysis or decreased vision from optic neuropathy is often the first symptom of the disease. Papillitis is usually absent in multiple sclerosis due to the more posterior involvement of the nerve.

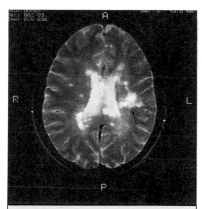

Fig. 61 Magnetic resonance imaging of the brain. Areas of high intensity correspond to demyelinating plaques, which are present in 90% of known multiple sclerosis cases.

The pupil

Both pupils are equally round and approximately 3−4 mm in diameter. Aniscoria refers to a difference in pupil size and 4% of normal people may have as much as 1 mm of difference. Miosis is a constricted pupil and mydriasis is a dilated pupil. Pupil size is determined by a dilator muscle controlled by the sympathetic nerve and a constrictor muscle that has cholinergic innervation via CN III.

Sympathetic nerve

The iris dilator muscle and Müller's muscle that elevates the lid are both stimulated by the sympathetic nerve that begins in the hypothalmus (Fig. 62) and descends down the spinal column. At C8 to T2 it synapses and then exits and passes over the apex of the lung. It ascends in the neck until it synapses, and follows the carotid artery into the skull and orbit. It dilates the pupil in response to the

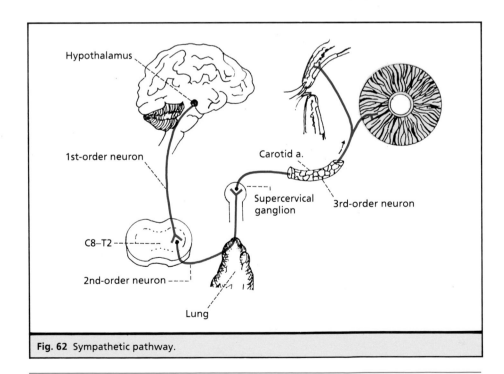

Fig. 62 Sympathetic pathway.

Causes of Horner's syndrome

Neuron I	Spinal chord trauma, tumors, demyelinating disease, syringomyelia
Neuron II	Apical lung tumors, goiter, neck injury, or surgery
Neuron III	Carotid aneurysms, migraine, cavernous sinus, or orbital disease

"fight or flight" stimulus. Damage to this nerve causes Horners' syndrome (Fig. 63): miosis, ptosis, and decreased sweating.

Pupillary light reflex (Fig. 64)

Light shining on the retina stimulates the optic nerve and then the optic chiasm and optic tract. Here, it exits from the visual pathway to stimulate the Edinger–Westphal nucleus in the midbrain. The pupillary fibers leave the nucleus and travel with CN III until it synapses at the ciliary ganglion in the orbit. It innervates the iris sphincter muscle. Light shining in one eye causes that pupil and the pupil of the other eye to simultaneously constrict. The latter is referred to as the consensual light reflex. Both pupils also constrict when the eye accommodates from distance to near. This normal state may be noted as PERRLA — pupils equally round and reactive to light and accommodation.

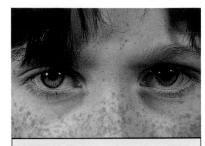

Fig. 63 Right Horner's syndrome.

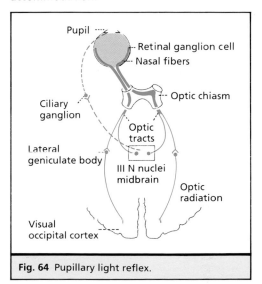

Fig. 64 Pupillary light reflex.

Causes of irregular pupils

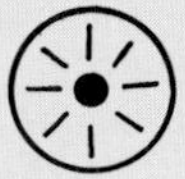

Miosis

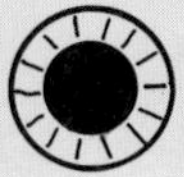

↑ Cholinergic

Pilocarpine and
phospholine
iodide drops
Morphine

↓ Sympathetic

Horner's syndrome
Aldomet
Reserpine

Irritation to
constrictor muscle

Iritis
Histamine release
from
inflammation

Mydriasis

↓ Cholinergic

Atropine
CN III paralysis
Adie's pupil
Antihistamines

↑ Sympathetic

Phenylephrine
Epinephrine
Anxiety
Cocaine
Decongestants

Damaged
constrictor muscle

High eye pressure
> 40 mmHg
Trauma especially
common with
hyphemas

Damage to the optic nerve (CN II) reduces direct pupillary constriction to light. The diseased eye will constrict well when light shines on the other eye due to the normal consensual reflex. Shining a light back and forth between eyes, called the "swinging light test" (Fig. 65), reveals the eye with optic atrophy to be dilating as the light shines on it since the stronger consensual reflex is wearing off. This is called a Marcus–Gunn pupil and is helpful in diagnosing optic neuritis. Also, in optic neuritis the patient claims the light is dimmer in the diseased eye.

Argyll Robertson pupil

In syphilis, the pupils may be irregularly constricted with a decreased or absent response to light, but a normal near reflex. The pupil dilates poorly with mydriatics.

Adie's pupil (tonic pupil)

This is a dilated pupil with a reduced direct and consensual light reflex. It reacts slowly to accommodation, and eventually becomes smaller and stays smaller than the other eye, hence the name tonic pupil. It is due to a benign defect in the ciliary ganglion. Resulting denervation hypersensitivity causes the tonic pupil to constrict intensely compared with the other eye in response to one drop of weak pilocarpine 1/10%.

Visual field testing

The field of vision of each eye extends to 170° in the horizontal and 130° in the vertical meridian. Routine testing of vision with a Snellen chart recorded as 20/20 only means that the central few degrees corresponding to the macula are normal.

1 Amsler grid. This hand-held black crosshatched card (as shown on the back cover of this book) tests the central 20° of the visual field. Hold the card at 14 inches and ask the patient if he or she loses the central white dot, continuity of lines, or the corners of the square. Waviness of lines is called metamor-

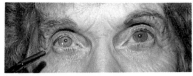

(a)

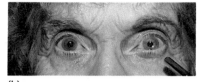

(b)

Fig. 65 Swinging light test. (a) Both pupils constrict when light shines in normal right eye due to consensual reflex. (b) Left pupil in eye with optic neuritis dilates as light shines on it, since consensual stimulation wears off.

phopsia, and is characteristic of a wrinkled retina from macular disease (Fig. 66).

2 A tangent screen is a sheet of black felt (Fig. 67). It measures the central 60° of field. The patient is seated 1 or 2 meters from the screen, with one eye occluded. The examiner moves a small white ball centrally until the patient first sees it. Areas blind to this small object are tested with progressively larger objects.

3 Hemisphere perimeters (Fig. 68) test the entire 170° of horizontal field and 130° of vertical field. Automated perimeters are expensive but save examiners' time. Static perimeters project increasingly intense stimuli at one location until it is first seen. Kinetic perimeters move a single intensity stimulus until it is no longer seen. Accuracy increases with the number of stimuli used.

4 Confrontation testing is used when instruments aren't available. The patient is seated opposite the examiner. The patient closes his or her right eye; the examiner closes his or her own left eye, and each fixates on the other's nose. The examiner moves an object in from the periphery and it should be seen simultaneously by both individuals.

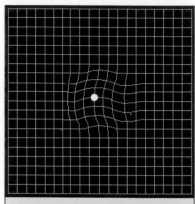

Fig. 66 Amsler grid. Distortion in macular degeneration.

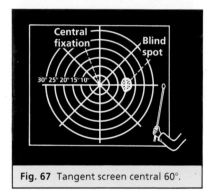

Fig. 67 Tangent screen central 60°.

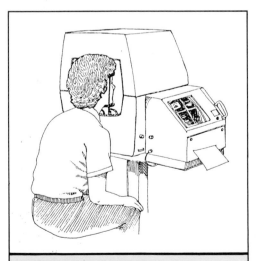

Fig. 68 Automated hemisphere perimeter tests central and peripheral fields.

Scotomas due to ocular and optic nerve disease

A scotoma is loss of part of the field. Relative scotomas are areas of visual field blind to small objects, but able to perceive larger stimuli. Absolute scotomas are totally blind areas.

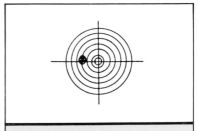

Fig. 69 Normal blind spot.

The normal blind spot is an absolute scotoma located 15° temporal to central fixation, which corresponds to the normal absence of rods and cones on the optic disk. It is plotted first (Fig. 69). If the blind spot cannot be located, the test is considered unreliable.

Central scotomas (Fig. 70) occur in macular degeneration. Central and paracentral scotomas (Fig. 71) are most characteristic of optic nerve disorders.

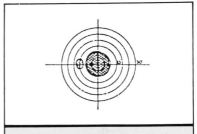

Fig. 70 Central scotoma.

Arc scotomas around central fixation are most typical of glaucoma (Fig. 72).

Unilateral altitudinal scotomas are defects above or below the horizontal meridian and are caused by an occlusion of a superior or inferior retinal artery or vein (Fig. 73).

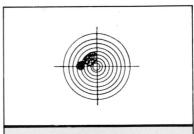

Fig. 71 Paracentral scotoma.

Scotomas due to brain lesions

Field defects help to localize the site of brain lesions. Light focused on the temporal retina passes through the optic nerve and stimulates the occipital cortex on the same side, whereas fibers carrying impulses from the nasal retina cross over in the optic chiasm and stimulate the brain on the opposite side (Fig. 74). Therefore, defects at or posterior to the chiasm cause loss of vision in both eyes. The scotomas respect the vertical meridian and are called hemianopic.

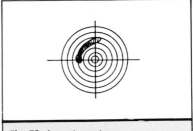

Fig. 72 Arcuate scotoma.

The term homonymous refers to having the same defect in both eyes. For example, right homonymous hemianopsia.

1 In the optic chiasm, the nasal axons from each eye cross over. Pituitary tumors press on these fibers and cause a bitemporal hemianopsia.

2 Optic tract lesions cause incongruous hemianopsia, i.e., unequal in each eye.

3 Optic radiation defects are often partial because the fibers are so widespread. A parietal lobe tumor damages the superior half of the left radiation causing a right homonymous inferior quadrantopsia.

4 Occipital cortex lesions usually cause a partial homonymous hemianopsia that is often vascular in origin, but tumors, trauma, and abscesses are also common.

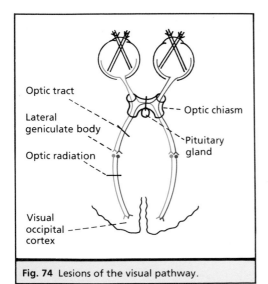

Fig. 74 Lesions of the visual pathway.

Altitudinal scotoma figure:

Fig. 73 Altitudinal scotoma.

Color vision

Color vision depends on the ability to see three primary colors: red, green, and blue. Partial defects are inherited in 7% of males and 0.5% of females using Isihara or American optical pseudoisochromatic plates. Loss of color vision could limit one's ability to become an electrician, airline pilot, or other profession requiring color discrimination. Acquired color defects may be due to retinal or visual pathway disease, the most common of which is optic neuritis. In acquired cases, test each eye separately, and look for differences.

Nystagmus

This is an involuntary rhythmic movement of the eyes in a horizontal, vertical, or rotary fashion. Pendular nystagmus means equal motion in each direction, while the jerky type has a quicker movement in one direction than the other.

Normal types

Optokinetic nystagmus is a jerky type of movement, as occurs when one watches scenery go by while riding in a car (Fig. 75).

End-point nystagmus is a jerky type occurring in extreme positions of gaze.

Vestibular nystagmus is due to stimulation of the semicircular canals of the ear, either by rotating the body or placing cold or hot water in the ear.

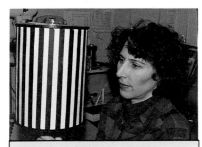

Fig. 75 Optokinetic drum that stimulates optokinetic nystagmus when rotated. Hysterics and malingerers faking total blindness cannot help but move their eyes.

Abnormal types

Gaze nystagmus occurs in certain fields of gaze. It is caused by drugs such as Dilantin or barbiturates, and in demyelinating diseases, cerebral vascular insufficiency, and brain tumors.

Congenital nystagmus is a pendular nystagmus starting at birth and usually causing reduced vision. If there is a position of gaze with less movement (null angle), eye muscle surgery or prisms may be tried to move this position to straight-ahead gaze.

Spasmus nutans is a unilateral or bilateral pendular nystagmus beginning at about 6 months of age and often ending by 2 years of age. It may be associated with head nodding.

Blindness that begins early in life may result in pendular nystagmus.

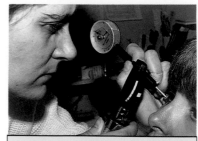

Fig. 76 Ophthalmodynamometry.

Circulatory disturbances affecting vision

Ophthalmodynamometry
(Figs 76 and 77)

This determines the relative pressure in the retinal arteries. Pressure is applied to the anesthetized sclera until the retinal arteries on the optic disk collapse. Differences of 20% in the two eyes is evidence for carotid narrowing on one side.

Intracranial aneurysms most often occur at arterial junctions in the circle of Willis. Pressure from an aneurysm at the junction of the carotid and posterior communicating artery (see Fig. 45, p. 21) is a common cause of CN III paralysis and is always associated with pain.

The cavernous sinus drains venous blood from the orbit and some of the face (see Fig. 45, p. 21). Carotid cavernous fistulas usually result from trauma and connect high-pressure arterial to low-pressure venous circulation. The results are a pulsating exophthalmos, an engorged conjunctiva, swollen closed lids, and a bruit over the eye (Fig. 78).

Cavernous sinus thrombosis (see Fig. 45, p. 21) results from an infection in the orbit, face, or tooth. Findings include lid edema, chemosis (conjunctival edema, see Fig. 146, p. 54), non-pulsatile exophthalmos, and decreased function of CN III–VI or the sympathetic nerve.

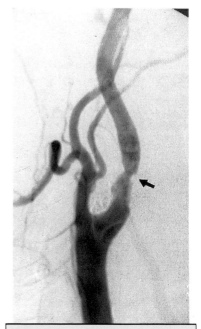

Fig. 77 Internal carotid artery narrowing.

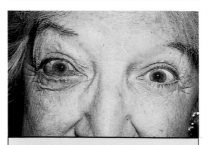

Fig. 78 Carotid cavernous fistula.

Arterial circulation to visual centers

(see Fig. 45, p. 21)

Blood supplied to the brain originates from the two carotid arteries in the anterolateral neck and the two vertebral arteries passing through the cervical vertebrae. Transient loss of vision in those persons younger than age 50 is often due to a migrainous spasm of a cerebral artery. This causes scintillating scotomas (Fig. 79), which are brief flashes of light and/or zigzag lines that may precede a headache. It may progress to a homonymous hemianopsia lasting for 15—20 minutes.

In elderly persons, transient visual loss is usually due to small emboli from arteriosclerotic plaques that temporarily blur vision as they pass through small vessels in the eye or visual cortex.

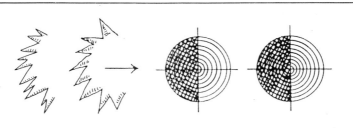

Fig. 79 Scintillating scotoma from migraine progressing to a homonymous hemianopsia.

Visual transient ischemic attacks		
	Carotid circulation	*Posterior cerebral circulation*
Cause	Cardiac abnormalities or carotid atheromas cause emboli to the retina (see Fig. 251, p. 88)	Neck disorders affecting vertebral artery or emboli from atheroma
Symptoms	Unilateral curtain lasting a few minutes (amaurosis fugax): rarely headache, confusion, contralateral hemiparesis	Hemianopsia in both eyes: usually history of headache, dizziness, diplopia, drop attacks, or ringing in ears
Tests	Angiography, ultrasound, ophthalmodynamometry, bruit over carotid artery in neck	Angiography
Rx	Anticoagulants or endarterectomy if >50% narrowing	Anticoagulants

External structures

Begin with the four Ls: lymph, lacrimal, lashes, and lids.

Lymph nodes

Lymphatics from the lateral conjunctiva drain to the preauricular nodes just anterior to the ear. The nasal conjunctiva drains to the sub-mandibular nodes (Fig. 80). Enlarged or tender nodes help to distinguish infectious from allergic lid and conjunctival inflammations.

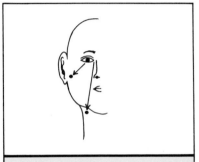

Fig. 80 Lymph drainage from the eye.

Lacrimal system

The tear film is made up of an outer oily component, a middle watery layer, and a deep mucous layer.

With most external eye infections, the tear film is highly infectious. In AIDS, only bloody tears are so far considered infectious. In any case, wash hands between examination of all patients.

With each blink acting as a lacrimal pump, the tear is moved nasally where it enters the

Type	Source
Oily	Meibomian glands at edge of eyelid
Watery	Constant secretion by conjunctival glands and reflex secretion by the lacrimal gland in response to ocular irritation or emotion. In this reflex, CN V is the afferent pathway and CN VI is the efferent pathway
Mucous	Conjunctival goblet cells

puncta and flows through the canaliculus, lacrimal sac, and the nasolacrimal duct (NLD) into the nose (Fig. 81). All eye drops are more effective and have less systemic side effects if patients press on the puncta and close the eyes for 60 seconds. This minimizes flow into the nose.

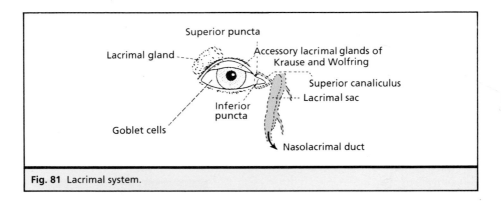

Fig. 81 Lacrimal system.

Dry eye

Tear production normally decreases with age and could result in a symptomatic dry eye (keratoconjunctivitis sicca). Patients complain of a gritty sensation with an occasional gush of tears from the lacrimal gland in response to the irritated eye.

The Schirmer test measures tears on the surface of the eye. A drop of anesthetic is instilled and a strip of folded filter paper is placed inside the lateral lid (Fig. 82). Less than 10 mm of moist paper in 5 minutes is presumptive of a dry eye.

Dryness may also result from medications such as anticholinergics, tranquilizers, antihistamines, and diuretics. It also occurs with collagen and rheumatoid diseases including Sjogren's syndrome (dry eye and mouth with arthritis).

Vitamin A deficiency is a leading cause of blindness in malnourished populations. The blindness results from a dry eye that causes corneal scarring and also from decreased function of the rod receptors in the retina, which

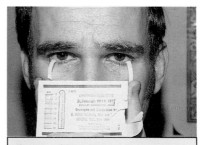

Fig. 82 Schirmer test.

requires vitamin A to make the visual pigment rhodopsin.

Dry eye is treated in the daytime with artificial tears and at night with ointments. In severe cases, the puncta may be closed with plugs or cautery to conserve tears. Room humidifiers may be tried.

Tearing

There are two causes of epiphora (tearing):
1 increased tear production due to emotion or eye irritation; or
2 normal tear production that cannot flow properly into the nose.

Once emotion and irritation are ruled out as the cause of tearing, an evaluation is made of the patency of the ducts leading into the nose. An obstruction is presumed if fluorescein dye placed on the conjunctiva (Fig. 83) disappears slowly and asymmetrically from one eye, or runs over the lid onto the cheek. Next, determine if the obstruction is in the puncta, canaliculus, or NLD.

Inspect the puncta for narrowing and be sure the puncta is not away from the globe as with an ectropion (see Fig. 105, p. 43). Rarely, the canaliculus may get obstructed due to an infection from *Actinomyces israelii*. In this case, incise the duct, remove sand-like concretions, and instill sulfacetamide drops. The canaliculus may also obstruct following lid injuries. To prevent this, tears of the canaliculus are repaired with a pigtail probe (Fig. 84), which is passed through the upper puncta to the torn lower canaliculus. Silicone tubing is placed on the tip of the probe and it is withdrawn back through the upper puncta. The probe is passed through the lower puncta and the other end of the silicone tube is put on the probe and it is withdrawn through the lower puncta. The skin is sutured (Fig. 85).

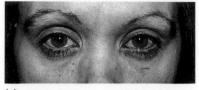

(a)

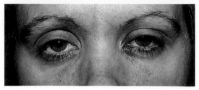

(b)

Fig. 83 (a) Fluorescein in both eyes. (b) Obstruction prevents exit of dye in left eye.

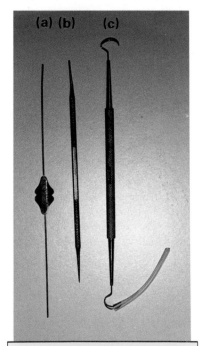

Fig. 84 (a) Punctal probe. (b) Punctum dilator. (c) Pigtail probe.

NLD narrowing in adults is common with aging or may be due to rhinitis. In infants, the end of this duct — the valve of Hasner — fails to open up at birth, and should be treated by 6 months to 1 year of age. In either case, irrigate through the puncta into the nose (Fig. 86). Resistance to irrigation confirms the diagnosis and is therapeutic if it washes out the obstruction or opens the valve of Hasner. If irrigation is unsuccessful a probe may be passed through the puncta into the nose (Fig. 87). If this still does not work, a temporary tube may be inserted for several months to stretch the duct. The final treatment is surgical creation of a new duct into the nose (dacryocystorhinostomy).

Besides tearing, NLD obstructions cause infections of the lacrimal sac (dacryocystitis, Fig. 88) due to stagnant tear flow. There is swelling and tenderness over the lacrimal sac with pus exuding from the puncta when pressure is applied to the sac. Rx: massage the sac; nasal decongestants; local and systemic antibiotics; treatment to open NLD.

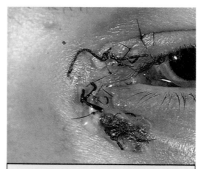

Fig. 85 Repair of canalicular tear.

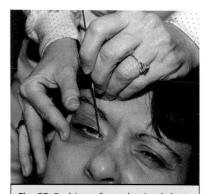

Fig. 87 Probing of nasolacrimal duct.

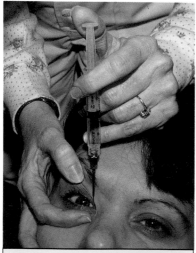

Fig. 86 Irrigation of nasolacrimal duct.

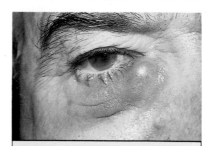

Fig. 88 Dacryocystitis.

Lashes

Trichiasis (inturned lashes) (see Fig. 136, p. 53) cause corneal irritations, and may be the result of an entropion (inturned lid), or trauma to the lid margin. Lashes can be epilated (pulled out), or the lash follicles can be destroyed with electrolysis or cyrosurgery.

Lice on lashes cause blepharitis and conjunctivitis (Fig. 89). Rx: Kwell shampoo.

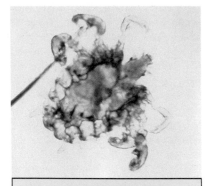

Fig. 89 Crab lice (*Phthirius pubis*) on lashes.

Lids

Lid swelling is commonly due to allergy, in which case the edema clears with a telltale shriveling of the skin between episodes (Fig. 90). Dependent edema caused by body fluid retention affects the lids on awakening and the ankles later in the day. Hypothyroidism (myxedema) and orbital venous congestion due to orbital masses or cavernous sinus thrombosis or fistulas are less common causes of edematous lids.

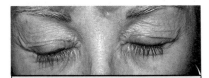

Fig. 90 Shriveled skin following allergy.

Dermatochalasis is loose skin (Fig. 91) due to aging, and is aggravated by recurrent bouts of lid edema. There may be palpable orbital fat that herniated through the orbital septum (see Fig. 116, p. 45). A surgical blepharoplasty is performed for cosmetic reasons or if resulting ptosis obstructs vision.

Lid-margin lacerations must be carefully approximated to prevent notching. Pass a 4-0 silk suture through both edges of the tough tarsal plate using the grey line for accurate alignment (Fig. 92).

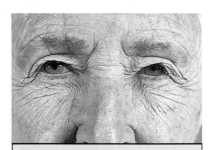

Fig. 91 Dermatochalasis.

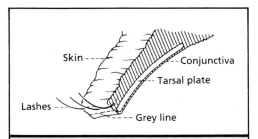

Fig. 92 Lid margin. The grey line delineates the mucocutaneous junction.

Cavernous hemangiomas (Fig. 93) appear at or shortly after birth and spontaneously regress by 2–3 years of age. Usually, they are a cosmetic problem, but may cause the lid to block vision. Intralesion injection of corticosteroids, excision, or radiation may be used if there is visual loss.

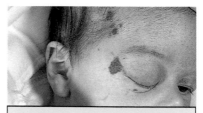
Fig. 93 Cavernous hemangioma.

Common skin conditions

The lesions in Figs 94 to 101 are electively removed for cosmetic reasons, while those in Figs 102 and 103 must be excised.

Xanthelasmas (Fig. 94) are irregular, yellowish, plaques on the medial side of the upper and lower lids. They are sometimes associated with hyperlipoproteinemia. Recurrence is common.

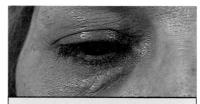
Fig. 94 Xanthelasma.

Verrucas (warts) (Fig. 95) are cauliflower-like growths of viral etiology; cauterize the base.

Molluscum contagiosum (Fig. 96) is small, smooth, round, dome-shaped, and centrally umbilicated. It is caused by a virus and resolves in several months. Curette rather than excise.

Seborrheic keratosis (Fig. 97), which is common with aging, is a benign, brown, rough-surfaced growth appearing stuck on like clay thrown against a wall.

Epidermoid inclusion cysts (Fig. 98) are intracutaneous benign, smooth, glistening, white balls filled with cheesy substance.

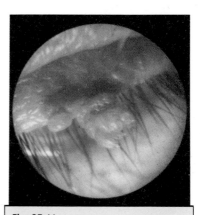
Fig. 95 Verrucas.

Nevi (Fig. 99) are benign, nonpigmented or pigmented, well-demarcated growths from early childhood. Suspect malignancy if growing, irregular edges, inflamed, satelites, irregular pigment, ulcerated, or bleeding.

Keratoacanthoma (Fig. 100) is a benign growth that resolves spontaneously. Rolled edges with umbilicated center filled with keratin makes it difficult to distinguish from squamous carcinoma, so a biopsy is often indicated.

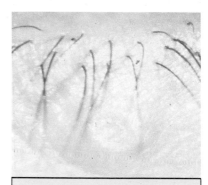
Fig. 96 Molluscum contagiosum.

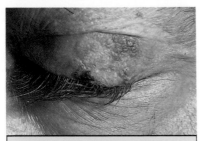

Fig. 97 Seborrheic keratosis.

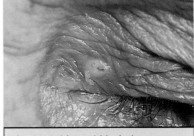

Fig. 98 Epidermoid inclusion cyst.

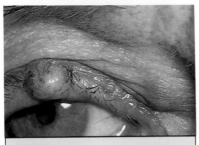

Fig. 99 Nevus.

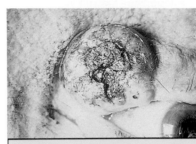

Fig. 100 Keratoacanthoma.

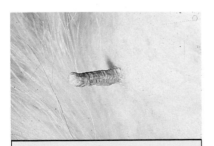

Fig. 101 Ingrown lash.

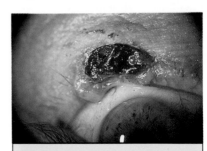

Fig. 102 Carcinoma.

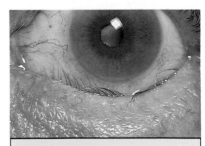

Fig. 103 Cutaneous horn.

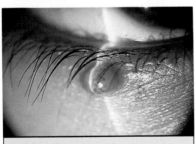

Fig. 104 Entropion.

Lashes commonly grow under skin causing a small cyst (Fig. 101).

The lids are a common location for basal, and less often, squamous cell carcinoma of the skin (Fig. 102). All chronic, hard, nodular, umbilicated, ulcerated, vascularized lesions demand a biopsy.

Cutaneous horns (Fig. 103) are keratinized overgrowths of seborrheic keratosis, verruca, or squamous or basal cell carcinoma, therefore a biopsy of the base is indicated.

An entropion (Fig. 104) is an inturned lid margin. It may be due to contraction of scarred conjunctiva, senile lid laxity, or spasm of the orbicularis oculi muscle. It is easily corrected with surgery.

An ectropion (Fig. 105) is an outturned lid often caused by senile relaxing of the lid that is aggravated in persons with tearing or taking eye drops, since they are constantly tugging or wiping their lids. Less common causes are CN VII paralysis or traction of scarred skin on the lower lid. Correct with surgery.

Myokymia (lid spasm) is a benign contraction of a few fibers of the orbicularis muscle. It usually lasts up to a few weeks and requires no treatment. Essential blepharospasm in which the eyes repeatedly close is more serious. The cause is unknown and it is treated with surgical destruction of the CN VII or injection of botulinum toxin into the muscle.

An epicanthal skin fold connects the nasal upper and lower lids (Fig. 106), and is common in infants and oriental persons. It gives the false impression of a cross-eye called pseudo-strabismus.

Ptosis is a drooping lid that rests more than 2 mm below the corneal margin. It may be congenital, or due to a CN III or sympathetic nerve paralysis, or laxity of lid tissue due to aging. It is often the first sign of myasthenia gravis, in which case the ptosis may worsen when tired, or after a provocative test such as asking the patient to look up for several minutes (Figs 107 and 108).

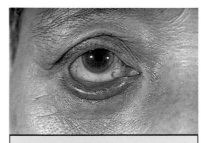
Fig. 105 Ectropion.

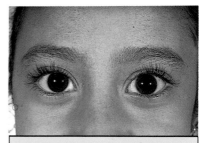
Fig. 106 Epicanthal skin folds.

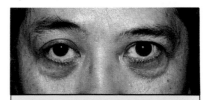
Fig. 107 Myasthenia gravis: no ptosis.

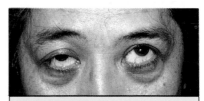
Fig. 108 Myasthenia gravis: ptosis after looking up for 5 minutes.

Blepharitis is inflammation of the lid margin with redness and flaking (Fig. 109). It is often chronic and may be associated with allergy, seborrheic dermatitis (dandruff), or acne rosacea (see Fig. 157, p. 58). Infection and ulceration may result in loss of lashes. Toxins from *Staphylococcus* bacteria can cause marginal corneal ulcers. Rx: routine cleansing of lashes with baby shampoo and/or topical antibiotic with or without steroid.

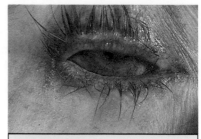
Fig. 109 Blepharitis.

Styes are pimples on the lid margin external to the lashes due to infection (Fig. 110). Rx: hot soaks, local antibiotics, incision. Systemic antibiotics are indicated if there is surrounding cellulitis.

Chalazions are internal to the lashes caused by infections of a meibomian gland on the lid (Fig. 111). They can become chronic granulomas. Rx: hot soaks, topical anesthetic, and sometimes local steroid. A chalazion may require incision and drainage.

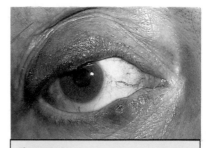
Fig. 110 Sty.

Lid cellulitis is a diffuse infection often due to a sty, chalazion, bug bite, or cut. Lids are red and tender (Fig. 112). There may be adenopathy and fever. Rx: topical and systemic antibiotics. Shriveled skin as in Fig. 90, p. 40, is an initial indication that lid cellulitis or orbital cellulitis is responding to treatment.

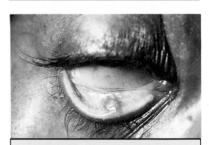
Fig. 111 Chalazion.

Orbital cellulitis causes the lids to be swollen shut (Fig. 113). The globe may not move (ophthalmoplegia) and there is chemosis, fever, adenopathy, and exophthalmos. It is most often due to sinusitis, but also occurs with facial or tooth infections. Rx: hospitalize the patient and treat with systemic antibiotics. Orbital cellulitis can spread to the cavernous sinus and cause thrombosis and death.

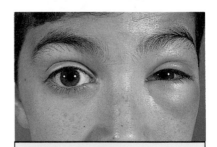
Fig. 112 Lid cellulitis.

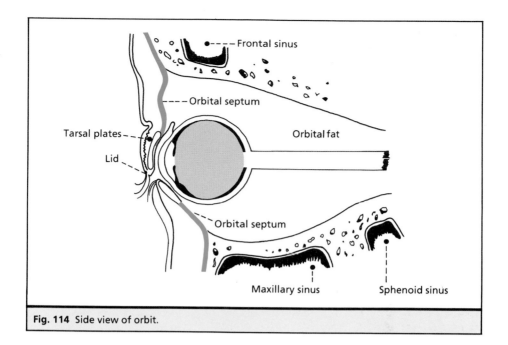

Fig. 114 Side view of orbit.

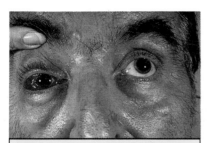

Fig. 113 Orbital cellulitis with chemosis and ophthalmoplegia causing inability to look up.

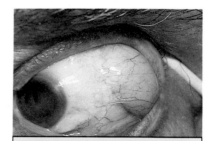

Fig. 115 Orbital fat under conjunctiva.

An orbital septum connecting the lid tarsal plates to the orbital rim (Fig. 114) acts as a barrier protecting the orbit from these common lid infections. Beware of the rare breakthrough. Orbital fat may migrate under the conjunctiva (Fig. 115) or herniate through the septum under the skin (Fig. 116).

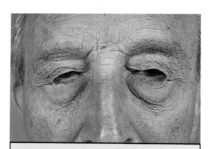

Fig. 116 Prolapsed fat through septum is palpable under skin.

The orbit

The orbit is a cone-shaped vault (Fig. 117). At its apex are three orfices through which pass the nerves, arteries, and veins supplying the eye.

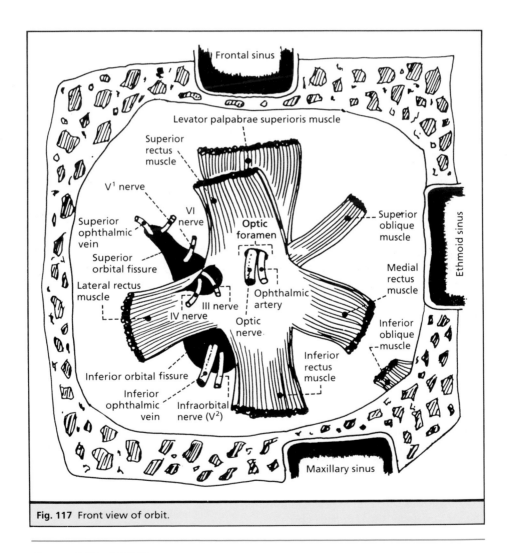

Fig. 117 Front view of orbit.

1 Superior orbital fissure: CN III, IV, VI, sympathetic nerve, and superior orbital vein.
2 Inferior orbital fissure: infraorbital (V^2) nerve, inferior orbital vein.
3 Optic foramen: optic nerve, ophthalmic artery, sympathetic nerve.

Around the optic foramen are the origins of all of the extraocular muscles except the inferior oblique, which attaches to the nasal portion of the anterior inferior orbit. The orbit is surrounded by four sinus cavities. This is important since infections can spread from the sinuses and cause an orbital cellulitis, and also because patients with sinusitis commonly present to an eye doctor thinking their pain is due to eye disease. The superior and inferior ophthalmic veins that drain the orbit and part of the face flow into the cavernous sinus and must be considered as a potential source for meningitis.

Exophthalmos

Exophthalmos (proptosis) is a protrusion of the eyeball caused by an increase in orbital contents. It is measured with an exophthalmometer (Fig. 118). In adults, unilateral and bilateral cases are most often due to thyroid disease. In children, unilateral cases are most often due to orbital cellulitis. Other causes are metastatic tumors, orbital hemorrhage, cavernous sinus thrombosis or fistulas, sinus mucoceles, or the following primary orbital tumors:

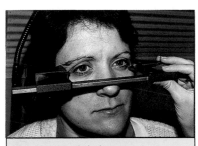

Fig. 118 Exophthalmometer.

1 hemangioma;
2 rhabdomyosarcoma;
3 pseudotumor;
4 lipoma;
5 dermoid;
6 lacrimal gland tumor;
7 glioma of the optic nerve;
8 lymphoma;
9 meningioma.

Enophthalmos

Enophthalmos is a retracted globe. The most common cause is a blow to the orbit that raises intraorbital pressure causing the thin roof of the maxillary sinus to fracture (Fig. 119). This is called a "blow-out" fracture. Associated signs may include subconjunctival hemorrhage, entrapment of the inferior rectus muscle in the fracture causing restriction of upward gaze, and vertical diplopia (Fig. 120). Hypesthesia of the cheek is due to infraorbital nerve damage. Rx: surgical insertion of silicone implant in the floor of the orbit if diplopia or enophthalmos persists.

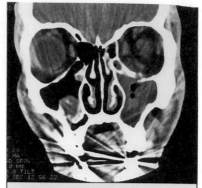

Fig. 119 Computed tomography scan of orbital blow-out fracture.

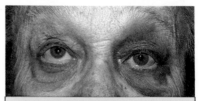

Fig. 120 Restriction of upward gaze due to blow-out fracture.

Slit-lamp examination and glaucoma

The slit lamp projects a beam of light onto the eye, which is viewed through a microscope (Fig. 121). The long wide beam is useful in scanning surfaces such as lids, conjunctiva, and sclera. The short narrow beam is used to study fine details.

Cornea

The cornea is the avascular, transparent, anterior continuation of the sclera. The corneal–scleral junction is called the limbus. A slit-beam cross-section of a normal cornea reveals, as keyed to Fig. 122,
1 anterior band epithelium on Bowman's membrane;
2 cross section through stroma;
3 posterior band endothelium on Descemet's membrane.

Corneal inflammation (keratitis) and abrasions are very painful because of the extensive number of corneal sensory fibers.

Corneal abrasions (Figs 123 and 124) due to trauma present daily with pain and a "red" eye. The de-epithelialized area stains bright green with fluorescein and a cobalt blue light Rx: topical cycloplegic (Cyclogel) 1% and a broad-spectrum antibiotic with a pressure patch (two patches) and oral analgesic. Most abrasions clear within 24–48 hours.

Topical proparicaine 0.5% anesthetizes the cornea within 20 seconds and lasts a few minutes. Never prescribe it for relief of pain since continued use damages the cornea. It is used to facilitate examination of a painful eye, prior to tonometry, and for removal of corneal foreign bodies. To remove a corneal foreign

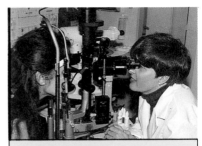

Fig. 121 Slit lamp.

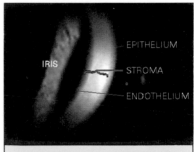

EPITHELIUM
IRIS
STROMA
ENDOTHELIUM

Fig. 122 Slit-beam cross-section of a cornea.

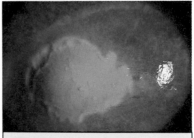

Fig 123 Corneal abrasion.

body, use a sterile needle and patch with antibiotics.

Keratoconus (Figs 125 and 126) is a bilateral central thinning and bulging (ectasia) of the cornea to a conical shape. It is associated with folds in Bowman's and Descemet's membranes. It begins between ages 10 and 30, often in allergic persons. The resulting irregular type of astigmatism corrects poorly with glasses and may require contact lenses or a corneal transplant that is successful in restoring reading vision in at least 90% of cases.

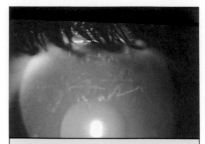

Fig. 124 Linear abrasions from trichiasis or particle under lid.

Corneal transplantation (keratoplasty) (Fig. 127) is used to replace an opaque or vision-distorting cornea with a donor cornea. Forty thousand operations a year are performed in the USA by ophthalmologists specializing in this procedure. There is a 90% success rate.

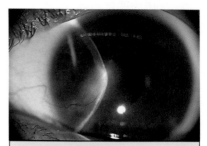

Fig. 125 Keratoconus.

Corneal ulceration is usually due to a bacterial infection, but occasionally viral and rarely fungal infection. It follows abrasions, blepharitis, or conjunctivitis. Over 50% result from contact lens wear. There is a white base of pus cells, with surrounding corneal edema and conjunctivitis. Treat vigorously on an emergency basis since it always scars and in the case of *Pseudomonas* may perforate within 1 day.

Marginal ulcers (Fig. 128) are most common and may be due to infection or an immune reaction to staphylococcal toxins from associated chronic blepharitis. Rx:. topical hourly broad-spectrum antibiotics and close monitoring.

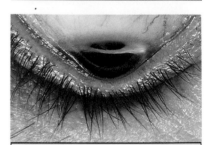

Fig. 126 Munson's sign: cornea indents lid when looking down. Courtesy of Michael P. Kelly.

Central ulcers (Fig. 129) are most ominous. Cultures are always needed with topical broad-spectrum antibiotics used up to every 15 minutes.

Hypopyon is a level of white blood cells in the anterior chamber, which is the space bounded anteriorly by the cornea and posteriorly by the iris and lens. It results from a sterile or infectious intraocular inflammation (endophthalmitis). Infectious endophthalmitis (Fig. 130) is a serious complication of intraocular surgery or a penetrating intraocular injury. A culture

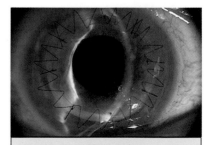

Fig. 127 Corneal transplant.

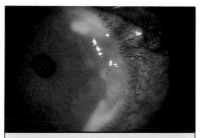

Fig. 128 Marginal corneal ulceration.

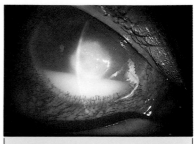

Fig. 129 Central corneal ulcer with secondary hypopyon.

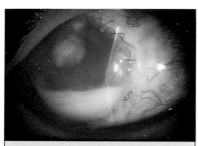

Fig. 130 Endophthalmitis with hypopyon following cataract surgery.

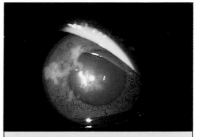

Fig. 131 Herpes keratitis.

of the aqueous and vitreous and topical, subconjunctival, intravitreal, and systemic broad-spectrum antibiotics are started immediately since blindness often results.

Herpes keratitis (Fig. 131) presents with a gritty ocular sensation, conjunctivitis, and an occasional fever sore on the lip. There may be small vesicles with central umbilication on the skin (Fig. 132). These often crust and then disappear within about 3 weeks. On the cornea, there are linear, branching lesions called dendrites that are almost impossible to see without fluorescein dye and a slit lamp. Herpes keratitis should be treated quickly since it usually scars and could penetrate the stroma causing a more chronic keratitis and iritis that might require the addition of topical steroids. Recurrences are common. Rx: trifluridine (Viroptic) 1% every 2 hours. Zovirax 200 mg p.o. every 4 hours may be indicated in resistant cases.

Localized superficial corneal edema (Fig. 133) has a translucent appearance, unlike an ulcer, which is opaque. In the common condition, called recurrent corneal erosion, a small patch of edema develops where the epithelium does not adhere well to Bowman's membrane. This often follows injury, but may be spontaneous. Patients awake in the morning with pain when cells slough off, usually just below the center of the cornea. The abrasion is treated with a patch and an antibiotic. The edematous epithelium is treated with hypertonic 2 or 5% sodium chloride solution (Muro 128 2% or 5%) in the daytime and sodium chloride 5% ophthalmic ointment (Muro 128 Ointment 5%) at bedtime. If sloughing continues, roughing up Bowman's membrane with a needle increases adhesiveness of cells.

Superficial punctate keratitis (Fig. 134) is diffuse epithelial edema, which appears as punctate hazy areas that stain with fluorescein (Fig. 135). Burning pain and conjunctival redness may result. Traumatic causes include improper contact lens wear, trichiasis (Fig. 136), rubbing of eyes, ultraviolet injury from a welder's torch, sunlamp, snow blindness, chemical injury, staphylococcal toxins, or a reaction to eye drops. Epithelial desiccation occurs with dry eyes or exposure associated with thyroid exophthalmos, overcorrection in cosmetic blepharoplasty surgery, or CN VII paralysis with inability to close the eye during the day or night (lagophthalmos) (Fig. 137).

Full-thickness corneal edema results from diffuse and severe damage to the epithelium or endothelium, which are both responsible for maintaining stromal clarity. Endothelium is commonly damaged from iritis or high eye pressure, and diffuse epithelial damage is often due to chemical injuries. There may be epithelial cysts called bullous keratopathy in severe cases (Fig. 138), or folds in Descemet's membrane (stria, Fig. 139). Corneal edema causes the patient to see halos around lights, which is a classic symptom of angle-closure glaucoma. Rejection of plastic lenses implanted during cataract surgery may cause permanent diffuse corneal edema and is one of the most common reasons for corneal transplant sur-

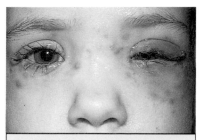

Fig. 132 Herpes dermatitis.

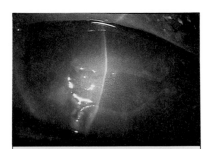

Fig. 133 Recurrent corneal erosion.

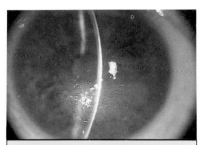

Fig. 134 Superficial punctate keratitis.

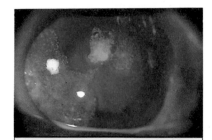

Fig. 135 Superficial punctate keratitis stained with fluorescein.

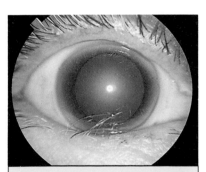

Fig. 136 Superficial punctate keratitis from trichiasis.

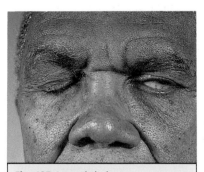

Fig. 137 Lagophthalmos.

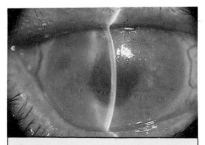

Fig. 138 Severe corneal edema.

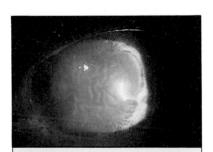

Fig. 139 Corneal edema with stria.

gery. Chemical injuries, with basic substances such as lye, are the most ominous since they immediately penetrate the epithelium and scar (Figs 140 and 141). Acid burns usually do not penetrate stroma or scar. Rx: irrigate.

Corneal vascularization is a response to injury. Superficial vessels are most commonly a response to poorly fitting contact lenses (Fig. 142), but also grow into areas damaged from ulcers, lacerations, or chemicals (Fig. 141). Deeper stromal vessels occur with congenital syphilitic interstitial keratitis.

Epidemic keratoconjunctivitis (Fig. 143) is a common highly infectious condition due to one of the adenoviruses that causes the common "cold." There may be a severe conjunctivitis lasting up to 3 weeks associated with photophobia, fever, cold symptoms, and an adenopathy. The main problem is the keratitis, which can last for months and, rarely, years. It does not scar but does restrict use of contact lenses until it clears.

Arcus senilis is a narrow white band of lipid infiltration separated from the limbus by a clear zone (Fig. 144). It occurs in almost everyone by age 80. Its occurrence in those younger than 40 warrants measuring blood lipids, which may be elevated.

Dermoid tumors (Fig. 145) are benign congenital growths often having protruding hairs. They are most common at the corneal limbus or in the orbit and may grow during puberty. They are removed if vision is threatened or for cosmetic reasons.

Conjunctiva

The conjunctiva is a mucous membrane. The bulbar conjunctiva covers the sclera and ends at the corneal limbus. The palpebral conjunctiva lines the lids. Fluid within the conjunctiva is called chemosis (Fig. 146) and is commonly seen in allergy and in rare cases of orbital venous congestion.

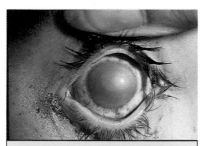

Fig. 140 Sodium hydroxide injury minutes later.

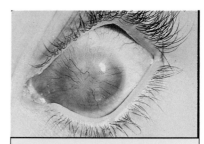

Fig. 141 Sodium hydroxide injury 3 months later.

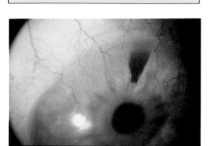

Fig. 142 Superficial vascularization often due to poorly fitting contact lenses. Courtesy of Michael Kelly.

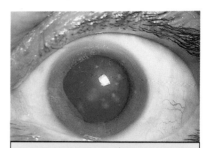

Fig. 143 Epidemic kerato-conjunctivitis.

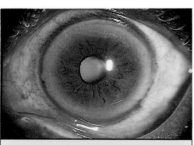

Fig. 144 Arcus senilis.

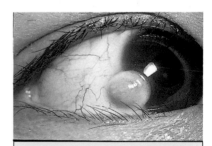

Fig. 145 Corneal dermoid.

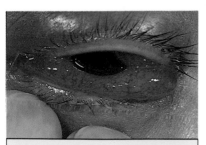

Fig. 146 Chemosis.

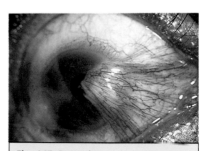

Fig. 147 Pterygium.

To examine the inner surface of the upper lid, first warn the patient, then "flip the lid" as follows:

1 have the patient look down with eyes open;
2 grasp eyelashes of upper lid at their bases;
3 pull out and up on lashes while pushing in and down on upper tarsal margin (patient should continue to look down during examination);
4 to return lid to normal position, have the patient look up.

A pterygium (Fig. 147) is a triangular growth of vascularized conjunctiva encroaching on the nasal cornea. Two causes are wind and ultraviolet light. It may be excised for cosmetic, comfort, or visual reasons. Recurrences of up to 30–40% are reported.

A pinguecula (Fig. 148) is a common, benign, yellowish elevation of the 180° conjunctiva, usually nasal but also temporal. It is composed of collagen and elastic tissue. It occasionally becomes red, especially with allergies (Fig. 149), and, rarely, may be removed if it is chronically inflamed, if it interferes with contact lens wear, or if it is a cosmetic problem.

Subconjunctival hemorrhages (Fig. 150) may be spontaneous, or result from rubbing of the eye, vomiting, coughing, elevated blood pressure, or, rarely, bleeding disorders. Recommend no rubbing, and no exercise or bearing down.

Conjunctivitis causes redness with a gritty sensation. Common causes are tired eyes, pollutants, wind, dust, dryness, allergy, or infection (Fig. 151). If there is pain, it usually indicates corneal or intraocular involvement. Vascularized elevations of the palpebral conjunctiva, called papillae (Fig. 152), are a reaction to an inflamed eye most unique to giant papillary conjunctivitis and vernal conjunctivitis.

Giant papillary conjunctivitis (GPC) is the most common cause for rejecting soft contact lenses. Large papillae develop under the lids which are an immune reaction usually to mucous debris on the lenses. Rx: change to disposable soft lenses or hard lenses. Keep lenses especially clean and decrease wearing time.

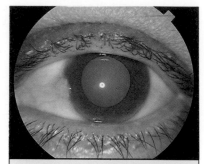
Fig. 148 Pinguecula.

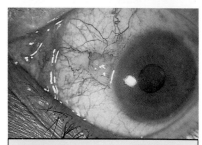
Fig. 149 Inflamed pinguecula.

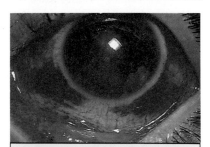
Fig. 150 Subconjunctival hemorrhage.

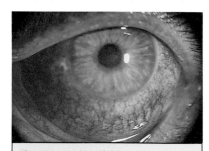
Fig. 151 Conjunctivitis.

Vernal conjunctivitis is an allergic condition in which large papillae under the upper lid abrade the cornea. It occurs in the first decade and may last for years. Antihistamine or steroid drops may be indicated.

White lymphoid elevations of the conjunctiva (Fig. 153) called follicles occur as a reaction to conjunctival irritation, especially from viruses, *Chlamydia*, and drugs. *Chlamydia* trachomatis causes two types of conjunctivitis.

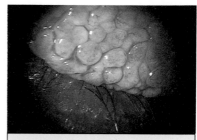

Fig. 152 Papillae of the palpebral conjunctiva.

1 Trachoma is a severe keratoconjunctivitis. It affects 500 million people worldwide and is a leading cause of blindness outside the USA. It begins with papillae and follicles on the superior palpebral conjunctiva. Conjunctival shortening may result in an entropion, which causes trichiasis. Inflammation of the cornea leads to superior vascularization (pannus), occasional corneal scarring, and loss of vision (Fig. 154). Rx: systemic tetracycline.

2 Inclusion conjunctivitis in adults is a follicular conjunctivitis with occasional keratitis. It is due to *Chlamydia* trachomatis — the most common sexually transmitted pathogen — and, therefore, must be ruled out more often in sexually active people. It is the most common cause of conjunctivitis in newborns who acquire it passing through the birth canal. Confirm with smear or culture. Rx: local tetracycline ophthalmic ointment and systemic erythromycin.

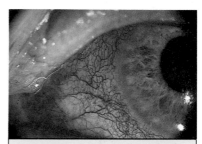

Fig. 153 Follicles of the palpebral conjunctiva.

Bacterial conjunctivitis often has a white–yellow discharge and is often due to *Staphylococcus aureus*, *Streptococcus pneumoniae*, and *Haemophilus influenzae*. It is usually treated without cultures (Figs 155 and 156).

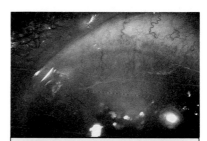

Fig. 154 Corneal inflammation from trachoma.

Eye drops commonly used for conjunctivitis because of their efficacy and low cost are chloramphenicol, sulfacetamide, and triple antibiotic (neomycin, bacitracin, polymyxin). Neomycin has a 5–10% incidence of allergy (see Fig. 6, p. 5); chloramphenicol rarely causes bone marrow suppression; and sulfur is static and will not kill *Pseudomonas*, which causes corneal ulcers. Therefore, some physicians prefer using gentamycin, Tobramycin and the new quinalones (Ciloxin, Chibroxin), or Polytrim (polymyxin and trimethoprim sulfate), which are all more expensive, but have fewer side effects.

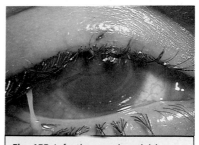

Fig. 155 Infectious conjunctivitis.

Chronic bacterial conjunctivitis, styes, chalazions, and blepharitis commonly occur in acne rosacea (Figs 156 and 157). This pustular dermatitis affects the forehead, cheeks, chin, and nose. Telangiectatic vessels and bumps, especially on the nose, are pathognomonic.

Viruses cause half the infectious cases of conjunctivitis. There is usually a watery discharge associated with "cold symptoms" and a preauricular node. It is often treated with antibiotics since it is difficult to be sure the infection is not bacterial and cultures are not usually practical. Antibiotic–steroid combinations may relieve symptoms, but could aggravate an atypical herpes simplex infection.

Allergic conjunctivitis is an intermittent condition associated with itching and slight redness. Signs include stringy mucous discharge, chemosis, and puffy lids. Treatment begins with avoidance of known irritants, discontinuing make-up, and applying cold compresses. Over-the-counter decongestants and zinc astringent drops are useful. Decongestant/antihistamine drops such as naphazoline/antazoline (Vasocon-A), relieve symptoms. Topical Cromolyn 4% (Opticrom) is another safe treatment that acts by inhibiting histamine release from mast cells. Acular (ketorolac) is a nonsteroidal antiprostaglandin drop used to treat ocular itching due to seasonal allergy. Steroids are most effective, but side effects limit their use. Medrysone 1% (HMS) is a steroid with minimal pressure-elevating effect. If treatment is prolonged with any drop, an allergist should be consulted.

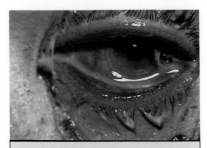

Fig. 156 Bacterial blepharoconjunctivitis.

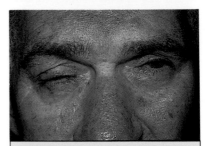

Fig. 157 Blepharoconjunctivitis in acne rosacea.

Conjunctivitis			
	Viral	*Bacterial*	*Allergic*
Onset	Acute	Acute	Intermittent
Associated complaints	Often sore throat, rhinitis, fever	Often none	History of allergy; nasal or sinus stuffiness, dermatitis
Discharge	Watery	Thick, yellow	Stringy mucus
Preauricular node	Common	In nonpurulent	None

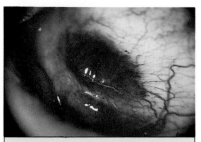

Fig. 158 Kaposi's sarcoma of conjunctiva.

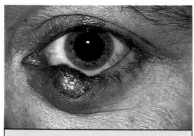

Fig. 159 Kaposi's sarcoma of skin.

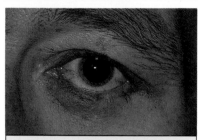

Fig. 160 Kaposi's sarcoma of skin (Fig. 159) treated with radiation. Courtesy of Jerry Shields.

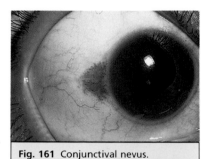

Fig. 161 Conjunctival nevus.

Kaposi's sarcoma (Figs 158–160) is a malignancy seen most often in AIDS. There is a nontender purple nodule on the skin or conjunctiva. Rx: radiation or excision.

Conjunctival nevi (Fig. 161) are common. Malignant transformation of nevi to melanomas is rare. Malignant transformation is suggested by satellites, rapid growth, elevation, and inflammation (Fig. 162).

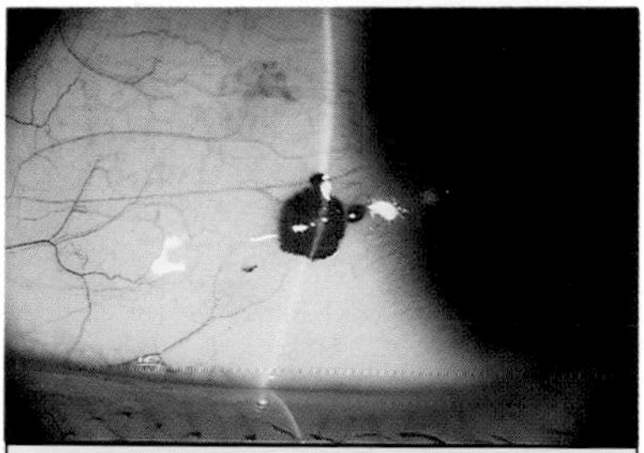

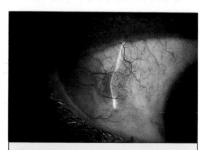

Fig. 162 Conjunctival melanoma.

Sclera

The sclera is the white, fibrous, protective outer coating of the eye that is continuous with the cornea. The episclera is a thin layer of vascularized tissue that covers the sclera.

Episcleritis is a localized, elevated, and tender inflammation of the episclera (Fig. 163). It lasts for weeks and may be suppressed with topical steroid if painful. It is a nonspecific immune response to surface irritants, but, infrequently, occurs in gout, syphilis, or rheumatoid arthritis.

Fig. 163 Episcleritis.

Scleritis is a severe inflammation of the sclera that may cause blindness. It is often painful and is most commonly associated with systemic immune diseases such as lupus erythematosis or rheumatoid arthritis. Anterior scleritis is associated with visible engorgement of vessels deep to the conjunctiva (Fig. 164). Posterior scleritis causes choroidal effusions and even retina detachments. Corticosteroids and anti-metabolite therapy are often required.

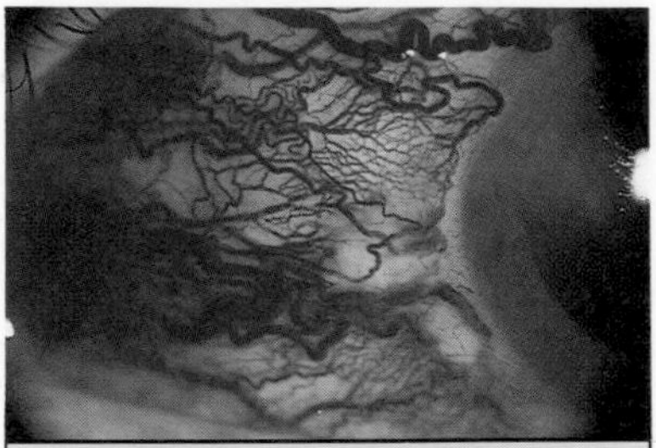

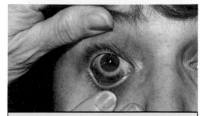

Fig. 164 Scleritis.

A blue sclera is due to increased scleral transparency, which allows choroidal pigment to be seen. It occurs normally in newborns, and abnormally in osteogenesis imperfecta, or following scleritis in rheumatoid arthritis, in which case the sclera is so thin it could rupture — scleromalacia performans (Fig. 165).

A staphyloma is a localized ballooning of thinned sclera in rheumatoid arthritis, high myopia, glaucoma, or trauma (Fig. 166).

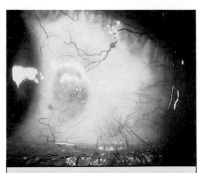

Fig. 165 Rheumatoid arthritis with thin sclera.

Glaucoma

Glaucoma is a disease in which elevated intra-ocular pressure damages the retinal ganglion cell axon that forms the optic nerve. The pressure impedes axoplasmic flow within the nerve, or reduces blood flow to the nerve (see Figs 55, 56, and 59, pp. 24 and 25).

Pressure is maintained by a balance between aqueous inflow and outflow. The aqueous produced by the ciliary body passes from the posterior chamber (the space behind the iris) through the pupil into the anterior chamber (Fig. 167). It drains through the trabecular meshwork and out of the eye through the venous canal of Schlemm.

Fig. 166 Staphyloma in rheumatoid arthritis.

Glaucoma vs glaucoma suspect

Normal intraocular pressure is 10−20 mmHg and should be measured at different times of day as there is a diurnal rhythm. Pressure greater than 28 mmHg should be treated to prevent loss of vision. Treat pressures of 20−27 mmHg when there is loss of vision, damage to the optic nerve, or a family history of

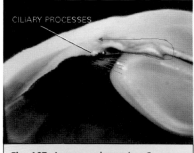

Fig. 167 Aqueous dynamics. Courtesy of Stephen McCormick.

glaucoma. Patients with pressures of 20–27 mmHg without these findings are called glaucoma suspects and are followed, but not treated.

A Goldmann applanation tonometer (Fig. 168) is the most accurate to measure pressure. It is used in conjunction with a slit lamp, and requires the use of anesthetic drops and fluorescein dye.

A Schiotz tonometer is a portable instrument (Fig. 169) that indents the anesthetized cornea and is used for bedside measurements.

The air-puff tonometer tests the pressure by blowing a puff of air at the eye. It is used by technicians since it does not require eye drops or corneal contact.

The iridocorneal angle

Aqueous exits from the eye through the trabecular meshwork (Fig. 170), which is the tan to dark brown band at the angle between the cornea and iris. The angle, normally 15–45°, can be estimated with a slit lamp (Figs 171 and 172), but a goniolens (Fig. 173) is more accurate. In open-angle glaucoma, the trabecular meshwork and the canal of Schlemm are obstructed, whereas in narrow-angle glaucoma, the space between the iris and cornea is too narrow so that aqueous cannot reach the trabecular meshwork. A narrow angle at risk of closing is graded 0–2. Angles of 3–4 are considered wide open with no chance of closing.

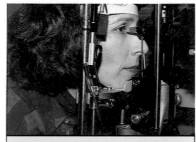

Fig. 168 Goldmann tonometer.

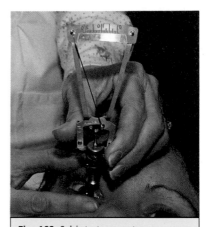

Fig. 169 Schiotz tonometer.

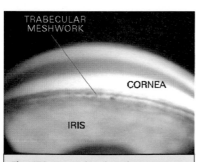

Fig. 170 Normal trabecular meshwork: grade 4 angle as seen with a goniolens.

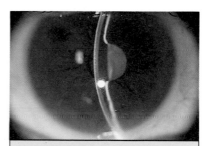

Fig. 171 Narrow angle in short hyperopic eye.

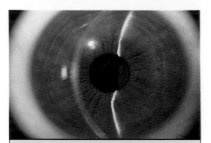

Fig. 172 Deep anterior chamber with wide open angle in long myopic eye.

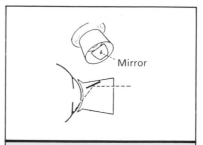

Mirror

Fig. 173 Trabecular meshwork seen with goniolens.

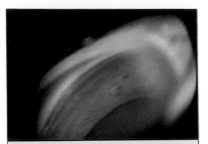

Fig. 174 Angle recessed posteriorly following traumatic hyphema. The recessed angle is seen as a wide dark band between the cornea and the iris.

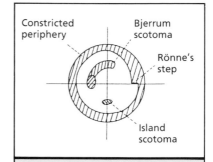

Constricted periphery

Bjerrum scotoma

Rönne's step

Island scotoma

Fig. 175 Visual-field defects in glaucoma.

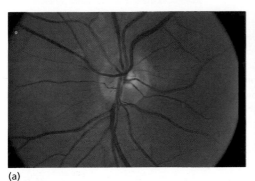

(a)

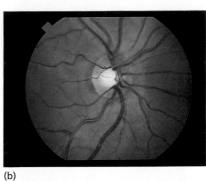

(b)

(c)

(d)

Visual field defects pathognomonic of glaucoma

(Fig. 175)

1 Bjerrum's scotoma extends nasally from the blind spot in an arc.
2 Island defects could enlarge into a Bjerrum's scotoma.
3 Constricted fields occur before loss of central vision.
4 Ronne's nasal step is loss of peripheral nasal field above or below horizontal.

Optic disk

In the center of the optic disk is a cup that is usually less than one-third the disk diameter, although larger cups can be normal. As the pressure damages the nerve (Fig. 176):
1 cup/disk ratio increases;
2 cup becomes more excavated and often unequal in the two eyes;
3 vessels shift nasally;
4 disk margin loses capillaries, turns pale, with infrequent flame hemorrhage (Fig. 176).

Therapy for open-angle glaucoma

The goal is to lower pressure below 20 mmHg, or at least to a level where there is no further loss of visual field or increase in cupping. It may require a combination of medications, one from each of the four categories on the following page, often given in the order listed. If maximum medical therapy does not control the pressure, argon laser may be applied to the trabecular meshwork (trabeculoplasty). If pressure is still too high, a surgical hole is created at the limbus (trabeculectomy) to drain aqueous through the sclera and under the conjunctiva (Fig. 177).

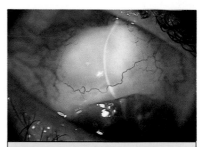

Fig. 177 Trabeculectomy: surgical fistula from anterior chamber to subconjunctival space.

Fig. 176 (*Opposite*) Optic cup/disk ratio. (a) C/D = 0.25; (b) C/D = 0.40; (c) C/D = 0.70 with hemorrhage; (d) C/D = 0.90.

β-adrenergic blockers	β-blockers decrease aqueous inflow and are the medication of first choice. Rx: usually 1 gtt b.i.d. Timoptic 0.25−0.5%, Betagan 0.5%, Ocupress 1%, and Optipranolol 0.3% may decrease heart rate and cause bronchospasm, so use cautiously with cardiac and respiratory diseases. Betoptic 0.25−0.5% has less pressure-reducing effect, but has less effect on the heart and lungs
Adrenergics	Propine 0.1% or epinephrine 0.5−2% decrease aqueous secretion and increase outflow. Rx: 1 gtt b.i.d. Ocular irritation, tachycardia, and increased blood pressure may occur. Avoid after cataract extraction, since 30% get macular edema, and in narrow-angle glaucoma, since it dilates the pupil
Cholinergics	1 Pilocarpine 0.5−8% increases the outflow of aqueous. Instilled q.i.d., usually starting with a 1% solution and increasing up to 4%. When surges of drug cause intolerable side effects, slow-release long-acting pilocarpine 4% ointment (Pilopine HS Gel) lasting 24 hours may be used at bedtime. A slow-release pilocarpine contact lens, Ocusert, lasts for 1 week 2 Echothiophate iodide 0.03−0.25% (Phospholine Iodide) used b.i.d. is a long-acting anticholinesterase. Browache and a small pupil often limit its use to the elderly after cataract surgery Local side effects of all cholinergics are cataracts, retinal detachments, browache, and a small pupil, especially troublesome at night
Carbonic anhydrase inhibitors	Acetazolamide (Diamox) decreases aqueous secretion, but gastritis, tingling extremities, and bone marrow suppression limits use. Dosage: 250 mg tab. p.o. up to q.i.d. or 500 mg sequel p.o. b.i.d. The i.m. or i.v. route is used when oral administration is impossible. An eye drop form of carbonic anhydrase inhibitor should be available soon

Angle-closure glaucoma

When the pupil of an eye with a narrow angle is mid-dilated, there is maximum contact between the iris and lens. Aqueous may not be able to flow from behind the iris through the pupil into the trabecular meshwork. Instead, this "pupillary block" causes the aqueous to be trapped behind the iris, pushing it forward against the cornea, resulting in total closure of the angle. The attack may be initiated by pupil dilators such as adrenergics, anticholinergics, stress, or a dark environment. There is a sudden elevation in pressure, often exceeding 60 mmHg. This pressure damages the pupil, causing it to remain fixed and dilated. Symptoms include pain, blurred vision,

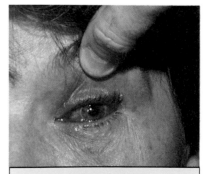

Fig. 178 Acute angle-closure glaucoma with dilated pupil.

halos, and nausea. Signs include a mid-dilated nonreactive pupil, corneal edema, and a reddened conjunctiva (Figs 178 and 179).

Treatment of angle-closure glaucoma includes Diamox, a β-blocker, and pilocarpine 1% drops with a hyperosmotic agent to lower the pressure so that the ischemic pupil will constrict and open the angle. When eye pressure must be reduced for short periods, mannitol 20% i.v. or oral glycerine 50% may be administered. Both draw fluid out of the eye by increasing the osmolarity of the blood. Once the attack is arrested, a laser iridotomy is performed (Fig. 180), which allows aqueous to flow into the anterior chamber and bypass the pupillary block. It is often a permanent cure.

Hyphema refers to blood in the anterior chamber. It usually results from a traumatic iris tear from its root on the ciliary body (Fig. 181). Complications include rebleeds, retinal damage, and glaucoma. Rx: bilateral patch and absolute bedrest for 5 days. Gonioscopy may reveal angle recession (see Fig. 174, p. 62) in which the iris insertion is shifted posteriorly, exposing a wide band of darkly pigmented ciliary body. Patients should be monitored indefinitely for glaucoma.

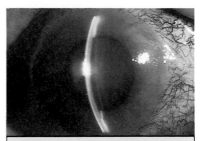

Fig. 179 Angle-closure glaucoma: shallow anterior chamber and corneal edema.

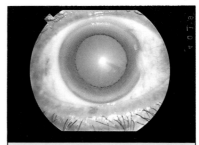

Fig. 180 Peripheral iridotomy at 2 o'clock.

Common types of glaucoma		
	Primary open-angle	*Angle-closure*
Occurrence	70% of all glaucomas	10% of all glaucomas
Etiology	Unknown obstruction in trabecular meshwork usually inherited; increases with age	Closed angle increases with age and hyperopia
Symptoms	Usually asymptomatic	Red, painful eye, halos around lights, nausea
Signs	Elevated pressure Increased disk cupping Visual field defect	Markedly elevated pressure Steamy cornea Fixed, mid-dilated pupil Conjunctival injection
Treatment	Usually eye drops	Laser iridotomy
Contraindicated medications	Corticosteroids	Pupil dilators such as adrenergics, anticholinergics, and antihistamines

The remaining 20% of all glaucomas have varied causes. Low-tension glaucoma causes loss of vision with pressure less than 20 mmHg, and is suspected when glaucomatous cup and field changes are seen with normal pressure. Secondary open-angle glaucoma is due to a blockage of the trabecular meshwork by pigment, hemorrhage, inflammatory cells in iritis, exfoliation from the lens, or scarring from rubeosis iridis. The trabecular meshwork may be damaged from traumatic tears as occurs with hyphemas, or covered with a membrane in the case of infantile glaucoma. One type of juvenile glaucoma is Sturge–Weber syndrome (Fig. 182) in which there is also angiomatosis of the face and the meninges with cerebral calcifications and seizures.

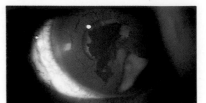

Fig. 181 Hyphema with large iris disinsertion (dialysis) from its root.

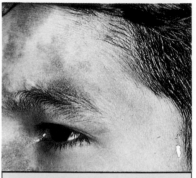

Fig. 182 Sturge–Weber syndrome.

Uvea

The uvea is composed of the iris, ciliary body, and choroid. All three are contiguous, highly vascular, and contain pigmented melanocytes. The ciliary body is made up of the pars plicata and the pars plana (Fig. 183). The pars plicata is anatomically the root of the iris. It comprises ciliary processes that secrete aqueous and the ciliary muscle, which focuses the lens by decreasing the tension on the zonules. The pars plana is the flat structure connecting the retina with the anterior segment at the ora serrata.

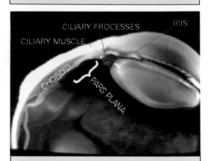

Fig. 183 Uvea. Courtesy of Stephen McCormick.

Malignant melanoma

A melanocyte tumor is the most common primary intraocular malignancy. It is unilateral and develops from the choroid in 85% of cases, the ciliary body in 9%, and the iris in 6%. Choroidal lesions are elevated and usually slate grey, but may be white to black with yellow–gold and uneven pigmentation (Figs 184 and 185) unlike a benign nevus, which is usually a more uniform grey color and flat (Fig. 186). This must be distinguished from metastatic carcinoma to the eye, which is also most common in the choroid but is usually lighter in color. Most often the primary site is the breast or lung.

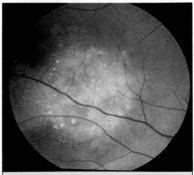

Fig. 184 Malignant choroidal melanoma.

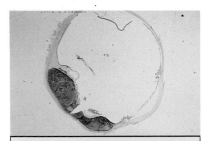

Fig. 185 Gross section of malignant melanoma.

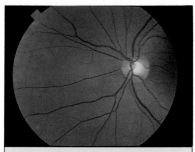

Fig. 186 Benign choroidal nevus.

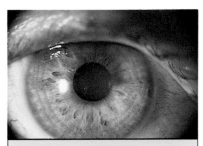

Fig. 187 Benign iris freckle.

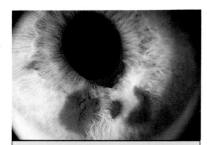

Fig. 188 Malignant iris melanoma with elevated lesions and distorted pupil.

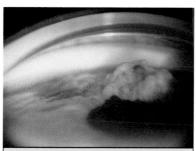

Fig. 189 Gonioscopic view of elevated iris melanoma. Courtesy of Michael P. Kelly.

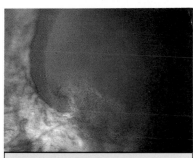

Fig. 190 Rubeosis iridis.

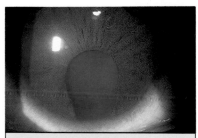

Fig. 191 Iris coloboma.

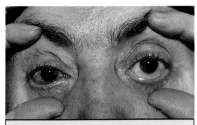

Fig. 192 Iritis.

Benign iris freckles (Fig. 187) and nevi are common, whereas malignant iris melanoma (Figs 188 and 189) is extremely rare. Lesions become more suspicious if they are growing, elevated, vascularized, distort the pupil, or cause inflammation, glaucoma, or cataracts.

Rubeosis iridis is a serious condition in which abnormal vessels grow on the surface of the iris (Fig. 190) in response to a central retinal vein occlusion, proliferative diabetic retinopathy, or carotid artery occlusive disease. Laser photocoagulation of the retina may cause regression of iris vessels. Untreated, the neovascularization causes a severe glaucoma.

An iris coloboma (Fig. 191) is due to failure of embryonic tissue to fuse inferiorly. It may also involve the choroid, lens, and optic nerve.

Anterior uveitis

This is an inflammation of the iris (iritis) and ciliary body (cyclitis). It causes ocular pain, tearing, and photophobia. Signs include miosis (small pupil), perilimbal conjunctival injection (Fig. 192), and anterior chamber flare and cells (Fig. 193). Flare refers to the beam's milky appearance due to elevated protein. With the slit lamp on high magnification and a short bright beam shining across the dark pupil, grade cells from barely visible (trace) to very many (4+).

Keratitis precipitates are deposits of inflammatory cells and protein on the corneal endothelium (Fig. 194). Cyclitis typically reduces eye pressure, since the ciliary body secretes the aqueous, but in severe iritis eye pressure may become elevated if cellular debris obstructs the trabecular meshwork.

Another complication of uveitis is posterior synechiae. These are adhesions between the iris and the lens capsule (Fig. 194). To prevent this, the pupil is kept dilated and steroids are given to prevent a fibrinous sticky aqueous.

Patients with juvenile rheumatoid arthritis and chronic iritis often develop a band of superficial corneal calcification known as band

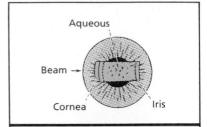

Fig. 193 Slit-beam view of flare and cells in anterior chamber.

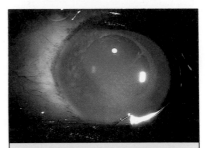

Fig. 194 Keratitic precipitates and posterior synechiae.

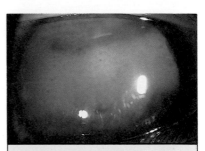

Fig. 195 Band keratopathy.

keratopathy (Fig. 195). It also occurs in sarcoidosis and hypervitaminosis D and may be removed with chelation.

Most often no cause can be found for iritis. Trauma or "flu" top the list of associated conditions. Less common causes are juvenile rheumatoid arthritis, ulcerative colitis, Crohn's disease, Reiter syndrome (young males with urethritis and conjunctivitis), ankylosing spondylitis (males with arthritis of lower spine), syphilis, toxoplasmosis, Lyme disease, 50% of those with sarcoidosis, or herpes simplex and zoster.

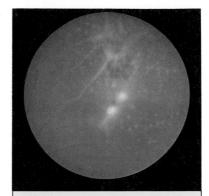

Fig. 196 *Toxoplasma gondii* choroiditis often reactivates next to old lesion.

Posterior uveitis (choroiditis)

(Fig. 196)

Posterior uveitis is characterized by white exudates on the retina sometimes obscured from view by cells extending into the vitreous. It leads to chorioretinal atrophy with pigment mottling (Fig. 197). Often no cause is found, but the following etiologies should be considered.
1 Bacterial: syphilis, tuberculosis.
2 Viral: herpes simplex, cytomegalovirus in 25% of AIDS patients.
3 Fungal: histoplasmosis, candidiasis.
4 Parasitic: *Toxoplasma, Toxocara.*
5 Immunosuppression: AIDS predisposes to several of above.
6 Autoimmune: Behcet's disease (mouth and genital ulcers with dermatitis); sympathetic ophthalmia.

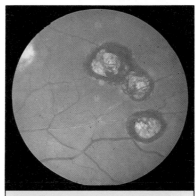

Fig. 197 Old toxoplasmosis scar: sclera visible through atrophic retina and choroid.

Sympathetic ophthalmia refers to a traumatic or surgical injury to the uvea of one eye causing an immune uveitis in the uninvolved eye. A penetrating injury involving the uvea is referred to as a ruptured globe (Figs 198–200). Handle the eye with minimal probing. Place the patient at rest with bilateral shields that exert no pressure and call the eye surgeon immediately. If uvea or retina are extruded from the eye and it cannot be repaired, the eye is often removed (enucleated). A silicone ball is then placed in the orbit and covered with conjunctiva (Fig. 201). A removable

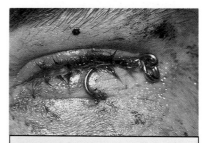

Fig. 198 Fish hook in eye.

scleral prosthesis painted to match the other eye is placed on the conjunctiva. Enucleation should be performed within 10 days of the injury to prevent sympathetic ophthalmia.

Treatment of any uveitis is directed at the specific cause if one is found. The inflammation is suppressed with topical, subconjunctival, or systemic steroids. An anticholinergic is used to decrease pain from ciliary spasm and for dilation, which prevents synechae from causing a permanently miotic pupil. The inflammation from posterior uveitis is treated with retrobulbar or systemic corticosteroids, especially when the macula or optic disk are threatened.

Local side effects of corticosteroids include cataracts, glaucoma, and activation of herpes keratitis. Systemic side effects include reduced immunity, osteoporosis, or exacerbation of diabetes or gastric ulcers. Choose the route of administration that transports the steroid to the site of inflammation with the least side effects.

Anticholinergics are used to treat anterior uveitis, to dilated the pupil for retinal examination, and to paralyze accommodation when refracting children.

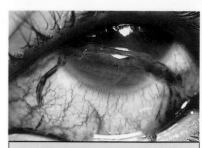

Fig. 199 Ruptured globe through sclera and cornea with prolapse of iris and ciliary body.

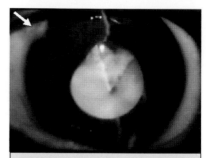

Fig. 200 Penetrating injury through iris and lens capsule with secondary cataract.

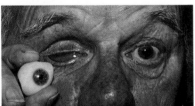

Fig. 201 Enucleated socket with scleral prosthesis.

Route	Steroid	Indications
Topical (drops or ointment)	Prednisone or Dexamethasone are most potent. FML or HMS are weaker with less pressure-elevating effect	Conjunctivitis, keratitis, scleritis, episcleritis, anterior uveitis
Subconjunctival	Celestone Soluspan	Severe anterior or posterior uveitis, endophthalmitis
Oral	Prednisone	Giant-cell arteritis, posterior uveitis, severe thyroid orbitopathy

Anticholinergic	Action time	Primary use
Atropine 0.5–1%	±2 weeks	Prolonged or severe anterior uveitis
Scopolamine 0.25% (Hyoscine 0.25%)	±4 days	Alternative when allergic to atropine
Homatropine 2–5%	±2 days	Anterior uveitis
Cyclopentolate (Cyclogel) 1–2%	±1 day	Cycloplegic retinoscopy; rapid onset (30 min)
Tropicamide (Mydriacyl) 0.5%	±6 hours	Often used with phenylephrine 2.5% for pupil dilation; rapid onset (15 min)

Vitreous

The vitreous is a clear gel made up of collagen fibrils. White cells in the vitreous (Fig. 202) are found in uveitis, endophthalmitis, or papillitis. Red cells are seen in vitreous hemorrhages, which occur most often with diabetic retinopathy (54%), retinal holes (17%), and retinal detachments (10%). Trauma may cause hemorrhages in a normal eye (Fig. 203). Fine reddish vitreous debris ("tobacco dust") liberated by the retinal pigment epithelium may be seen with a slit lamp and should alert one to a possible retinal hole or detachment.

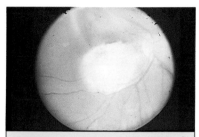

Fig. 202 Hazy view of toxoplasmosis choroiditis due to white cells in the vitreous.

The vitreous normally shrinks and liquifies with aging. This may cause a posterior vitreous detachment (Fig. 204) and fibrillar opacities to form within the vitreous. Patients complain of shifting cobweb-like floaters in their field of vision. As the vitreous shrinks, it may create traction on the retina especially where it is normally adherent to retina near the ora serrata and macula. This may cause a retinal hole and subsequent detachment. Therefore, in all patients with recent onset of floaters, a dilated retina examination is required. Less common causes of floaters are asteroid hyalosis (Fig. 205) and synchysis scintillans in which yellow spheres of calcium soaps are suspended in the vitreous. Ophthalmoscopically both of these appear like stars in the galaxy and are benign, requiring no treatment.

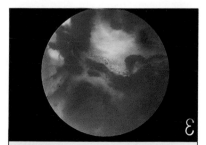

Fig. 203 Blunt trauma causing retinal hemorrhage referred to as commotio retinae. Hemorrhage may extend into vitreous.

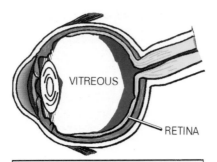

VITREOUS

RETINA

Fig. 204 Posterior vitreous detachment.

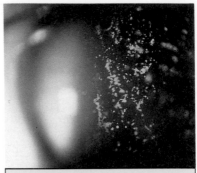

Fig. 205 Slit-lamp view of asteroid hyalosis with lens seen on left and vitreous on right.

B-scan ultrasound may be used to determine the status of the retina when a vitreous hemorrhage or cloudy lens and cornea obscure the view.

A-scan ultrasound measures the length of the eye. This length, together with the corneal curvature as determined with a keratometer, is used to calculate the power of the intraocular lens implant used in cataract surgery.

Cataracts

The lens consists of an outside capsule surrounding a soft cortical substance and a hard inner nucleus (Fig. 206). A cataract is a cloudy lens. It should be suspected when the patient complains of blurry vision and there is a hazy view of the retina with an ophthalmoscope. The diagnosis is confirmed with a slit lamp and described in one of the following ways.
1 By etiology: usually aging, but may be hastened by steroids, radiation, ultraviolet light, diabetes, and trauma (especially perforation of capsule, see Fig. 200, p. 70). The incidence is double in cigarette smokers.
2 By age of onset: congenital, juvenile, adult, senile.
3 By location in lens: cortex (Fig. 207), nucleus, or posterior subcapsule (often due to steroids, Fig. 208).
4 By color or pattern: cuneiform (spokes); zonular congenital type, involves one layer usually in or around the nucleus, and is often nonprogressive (Fig. 209); Brunescent (brown),

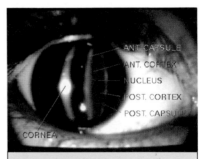

ANT. CAPSULE
ANT. CORTEX
NUCLEUS
POST. CORTEX
POST. CAPSULE
CORNEA

Fig. 206 Slit-lamp view of lens.

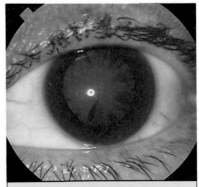

Fig. 207 Anterior cortical spokes (cuneiform).

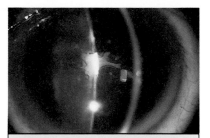

Fig. 208 Posterior subcapsular cataract.

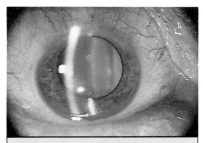

Fig. 210 Brunescent cataract.

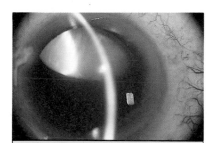

Fig. 212 Dislocated lens.

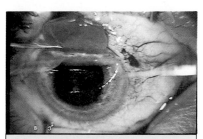

Fig. 214 Removal of hard nucleus in one piece. Courtesy of Richard Tipperman and Stephen Lichtenstein.

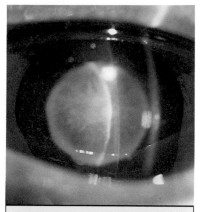

Fig. 209 Congenital (zonular) cataract surrounded by clear cortex.

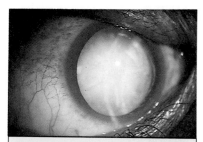

Fig. 211 Mature lens dislocated into the anterior chamber obscuring pupil and iris.

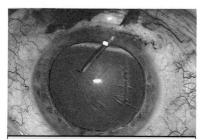

Fig. 213 Anterior capsulotomy: 50 punctures of anterior capsule prior to removal. Courtesy of Richard Tipperman and Stephen Lichtenstein.

often hard and difficult to break up with phacoemulsification (Fig. 210).

A cataract raises two questions. Is it responsible for the decreased vision? Is it ripe? Ripe is the layman's term for whether surgery is indicated. In most cases, a surgeon waits for a reduction in vision of 20/50 or worse, but indications vary with the patient's needs. Surgery is usually elective except in the case of a mature lens that might rupture or is already leaking (Fig. 211) or a dislocated lens in imminent danger of dropping into the vitreous or anterior chamber. Lens dislocation (Fig. 212) is due to rupture of the zonules. It occurs with trauma or may be associated with Marfan's disease, homocystinuria, or syphilis.

Cataract surgery is usually performed as an out-patient procedure using local anesthesia. The cornea is entered with a knife and the anterior lens capsule is removed (Fig. 213). The hard nucleus is either extracted in one piece (Fig. 214) or liquified with a phacoemulsifier, which has a tip that vibrates 40 000 times per second (Fig. 215). The advantage of phacoemulsification is that it causes a smaller wound, while its disadvantage is that it is difficult to perform and that the large amount of energy needed to emulsify a hard nucleus could damage the cornea or delicate posterior capsule. After the nucleus is removed by either method, the soft cortex is aspirated (Fig. 216). An intraocular lens is then inserted behind the iris in the remaining posterior capsule (Figs 217 and 218) unless the posterior capsule is torn in which case the lens is placed

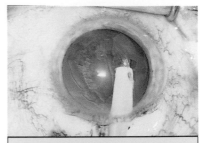

Fig. 215 Removal of soft nucleus by phacoemulsification. Courtesy of Richard Tipperman and Stephen Lichtenstein.

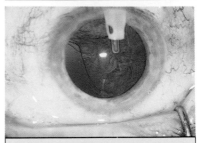

Fig. 216 Irrigation and aspiration of cortex. Courtesy of Richard Tipperman and Stephen Lichtenstein.

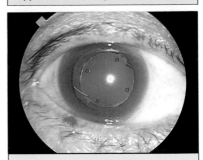

Fig. 217 Posterior chamber lens behind iris: preferred location.

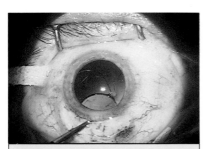

Fig. 218 Insertion of implant. Courtesy of Richard Tipperman and Stephen Lichtenstein.

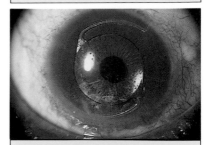

Fig. 219 Anterior chamber lens sometimes used when the posterior capsule is damaged during surgery.

in front of the iris (Fig. 219) — a location associated with more complications. This posterior capsule opacifies months to years later in 30% of cases and is called a secondary cataract (Fig. 220). It may be opened with a YAG laser (Fig. 221). A lens implant is inserted in 97% of cataract surgeries in which case the eye is referred to as pseudophakic. An eye is aphakic if no lens implant was used.

In aphakic eyes, a spectacle lens of about +12.0 D is required to focus the eye. It magnifies the image 33% larger than the normal eye, so that the two eyes cannot fuse, thereby forcing the patient to use one eye at a time. A contact lens that magnifies the image to a lesser degree than a spectacle lens can minimize the problem of image size disparity (aniseikonia), and allows binocular vision. However, contact lenses are often impractical with elderly patients.

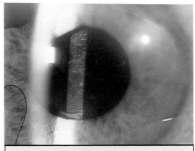

Fig. 220 Secondary cataract. Courtesy of Richard Tipperman and Stephen Lichtenstein.

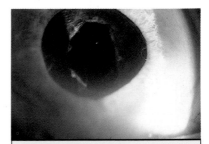

Fig. 221 YAG laser capsulotomy for secondary cataract of posterior capsule. Courtesy of Richard Tipperman and Stephen Lichtenstein.

The retina

Retinal anatomy

The retina is the sensory layer of the eye extending from the optic disk to the ora serrata (Figs 222 and 223, see also Fig. 260, p. 91).

Light stimulates the receptor cells called rods and cones, which transmit the message to the ganglion cell on the retinal surface. The long ganglion cell axons make up the optic nerve, which synapses in the brain.

The macula

The macula is rich in cones and is the most sensitive area of the retina. The retinal vessels terminate at its margin, and in its center is a pit called the fovea, which produces a bright reflex. The fovea has the most dense concentration of cones and is responsible for the most acute vision. This reflex decreases with age, and its absence in a young individual with a visual disturbance could indicate a macular dysfunction. When the macula is destroyed, the best corrected vision is 20/200.

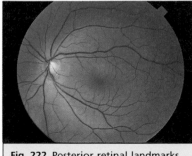

Fig. 222 Posterior retinal landmarks.

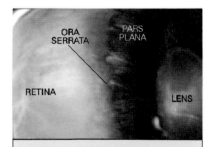

Fig. 223 Gross section of peripheral retina.

The optic disk

The optic disk is normally orange–red with a yellow cup at its center. The retinal artery and vein pass through the optic cup and bifurcate on the surface of the disk. Proliferated retinal pigment epithelium at the disk margin is also a normal finding (Fig. 224).

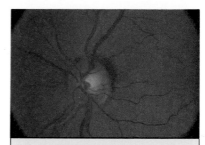

Fig. 224 Normal tigroid fundus with pigment around disk.

In axial myopia, the eye is increased in length and the retina may be dragged away from the optic disk margin, exposing the sclera. This is called a myopic conus or crescent (Fig. 225). In extremely myopic eyes often greater than 10 D, the retina is stretched so thin that it is absent in some areas causing a loss of vision. There may be hemorrhage at the macula called a Fuchs' spot (Fig. 226).

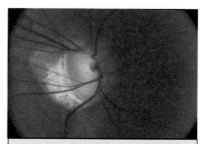

Fig. 225 Normal myopic conus (crescent) at disk margin.

Another disk variation occurs when the myelin sheath that normally covers the optic nerve extends onto the retina, appearing like white flame-shaped patches obscuring the disk margin. It is benign (Fig. 227). The disk margin may also be obscured by drusen (Fig. 228), which are small, round, translucent bodies. They may damage nerve fibers and cause an enlarged blind spot.

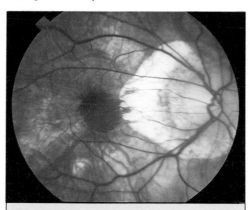

Fig. 226 Myopic degeneration.

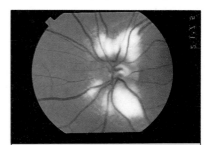

Fig. 227 Myelination of the optic nerve.

The choroid

The choroid is highly vascularized and nourishes the rod and cone layer and the retinal pigment epithelium. Unlike the tree-like branching of the retinal vessels, the choroidal

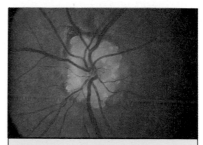

Fig. 228 Disk drusen.

circulation forms a criss-crossing network. As the retinal pigment epithelium loses pigment with age, the choroidal vasculature becomes more visible resulting in a tigroid appearance (Fig. 224).

Fundus examination

The fundus refers to the inner part of the eye seen with ophthalmoscopy, i.e., the retina, choroid, and disk. It is evaluated by first focusing on the optic disk and then on the retinal blood vessels and surrounding retina. The macula is examined last to minimize miosis and discomfort.

A direct ophthalmoscope (Fig. 229) allows for monocular visualization of the posterior half of the fundus where most retinal pathology is located. Use a negative lens for myopic eyes, and a plus lens for hyperopic eyes.

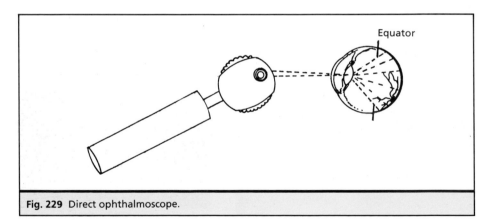

Fig. 229 Direct ophthalmoscope.

A binocular indirect ophthalmoscope (Fig. 230) consists of a powerful light source worn over the head and a hand-held lens, which allows the entire retina to be seen in three dimensions. Retinal holes and detachments at the ora serrata can be viewed by indenting the sclera with a small thimble worn on the index finger.

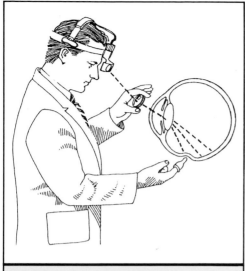

Fig. 230 Indirect ophthalmoscope.

A three-mirror contact lens (Fig. 231) used with a slit lamp gives a stereoscopic detailed view of the entire retina. It is useful in studying subtle changes in each layer of the retina, and to gauge optic cupping. Its disadvantage is the need for anesthetic drops and a solution on the eye.

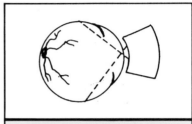

Fig. 231 Three-mirror contact lens.

Fluorescein angiography

(Figs 232–234)

Fluorescein dye is injected intravenously. As it passes through the retinal circulation, fundus photographs are made in a rapid sequence. This test is useful for evaluating retinal circulation. It demonstrates rate of flow, leakage from capillaries, staining of tissues, areas of nonperfusion, and neovascularization. Normally retinal blood vessels do not leak.

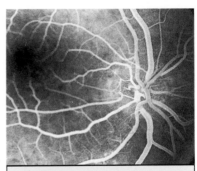

Fig. 232 Normal fluorescein angiogram.

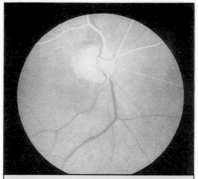
Fig. 233 Fluorescein angiogram of inferior retinal artery occlusion showing lack of perfusion inferiorly after 15.4 seconds.

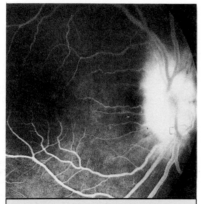
Fig. 234 Fluorescein angiogram of papilledema with leakage of dye from disk.

Papilledema (choked disk)

Papilledema is swelling of the optic disk usually due to increased intracranial pressure, in which case it is eventually bilateral. Unilateral cases are due to increased pressure in one orbit sometimes caused by a tumor. It begins with blurred disk margins and engorged disk veins. As it progresses, flame-shaped hemorrhages and cotton-wool spots develop in the peripapillary area (Fig. 235). Chronic, elevated intracranial pressure inevitably destroys the optic nerve resulting in optic atrophy.

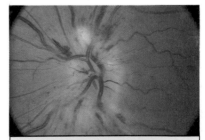
Fig. 235 Papilledema with elevated disk, engorged veins, and flame-shaped hemorrhages.

In 80% of normal eyes, there are subtle pulsations of the retinal veins as they exit from the globe at the optic cup. If pulsations are not visible they can almost always be elicited by exerting slight pressure on the globe (through the lid). In papilledema, one cannot see spontaneous or elicited venous pulsations. Swelling of the optic disk damages the surrounding retina and enlarges the blindspot, which helps confirm the diagnosis (Fig. 236). Elevated intracranial pressure that causes papilledema may also cause headache, nausea, and pressure on the CN VI resulting in diplopia.

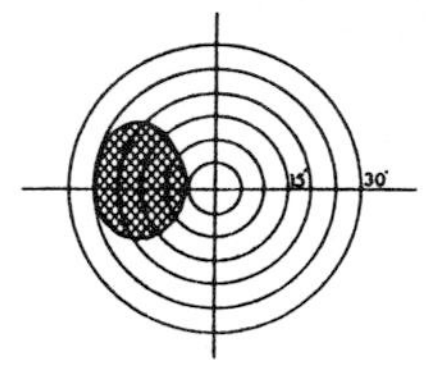

Fig. 236 Enlarged blind spot.

Differential diagnosis of papilledema

A swollen disk caused by optic neuritis (see Fig. 60, p. 25) is associated with a Marcus-Gunn pupil and loss of vision, whereas in papilledema the pupil is normal and there is usually no loss of visual acuity unless edema extends to the macula, sometimes resulting in a macular star (Fig. 237).

Early papilledema may be difficult to distinguish from drusen of the disk (see Fig. 228, p. 77) and myelinated nerve fibers (see Fig. 227, p. 77). All three blur the margin and cause an enlarged blind spot (see Fig. 236). On fluorescein angiography, however, only papilledema has leakage of dye (Fig. 234). A hyperopic eye might have a small disk with blurred margin but there is no leakage with fluorescein angiography. Like papilledema, central retinal vein occlusion (see Fig. 247, p. 87) may have venous engorgement, a blurred disk margin, and cotton-wool spots. In central retinal vein occlusion, however, the flame hemorrhages extend out to the periphery and there is usually more loss of vision. Malignant systemic hypertension can also cause a papilledema-like retinal appearance, which is easily distinguished by measuring blood pressure on all patients with blurred disk margins (see Fig. 245, p. 84).

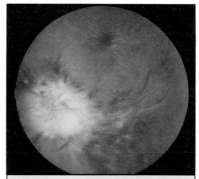

Fig. 237 Papilledema with macular star.

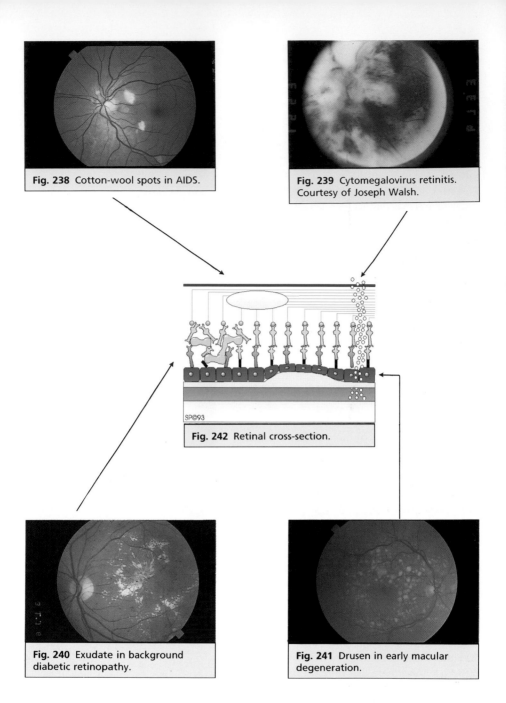

Fig. 238 Cotton-wool spots in AIDS.

Fig. 239 Cytomegalovirus retinitis. Courtesy of Joseph Walsh.

Fig. 242 Retinal cross-section.

Fig. 240 Exudate in background diabetic retinopathy.

Fig. 241 Drusen in early macular degeneration.

White retinal lesions

(Figs 238–242, p. 82)

Cotton wool spots (Fig. 238)

Ischemia of the superficial nerve fiber layer causes white, cloud-like lesions around the disk that obscure underlying retina. Causes include diabetes (see Fig. 256, p. 90), hypertension (see Fig. 245, p. 84), and papilledema. AIDS may have noninfectious retinal microangiopathy causing cotton-wool spots.

Inflammatory cells (Fig. 239)

White blood cells occur in posterior choroiditis (see Fig. 196, p. 69), retinitis, vasculitis (see Fig. 244, p. 82), or optic neuritis. They are irregularly shaped and often there is an unclear view because of overlying vitritis. Cytomegalovirus necrotizing retinitis occurs in 25% of AIDS patients mainly in late stages, and is rapidly blinding if untreated. Culture of blood, urine, or lungs confirms diagnosis. Rx: intravenous ganciclovir or foscarnet.

Hard (waxy) exudate (Fig. 240)

Leaking fluid from vessels leave behind a waxy, yellowish proteinaceous residue. It is seen most often in diabetes, but also in papilledema (see Fig. 237, p. 81) and hypertension.

Drusen (Fig. 241 and 261)

This is a hyaline thickening of Bruch's membrane of the retina (do not confuse with disk drusen). These are round, dull white, bilateral, and uniformly distributed, unlike asymmetric, yellow, irregular, waxy exudates. Drusen may progress to macular degeneration.

Retinal vessel disease

Retinal vessel walls are normally transparent. The vessels are visualized because of the blood within them. In arteriosclerosis, as the vessel walls become hyalinized they develop a dull "copper wire" and then a "silver wire" reflex and the relative thickness of artery to vein decreases (Fig. 243). At their junctions, the arteries and veins share a common sheath. Thickening of the arteriole causes indentation of the venule, referred to as A-V nicking (Fig. 243) inferior to the disk. This can lead to a retinal vein occlusion as shown.

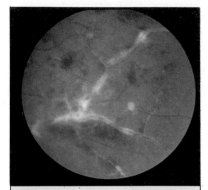

Fig. 244 Sarcoidosis with vasculitis causing "candle-wax" drippings on vessels. Courtesy of Joseph Walsh.

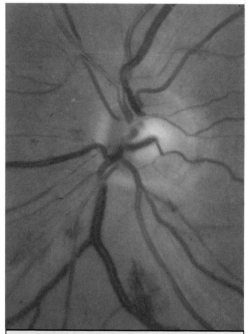

Fig. 243 Arteriosclerosis with partial vein occlusion demonstrated by engorged vein inferiorly and a secondary flame hemorrhage. "Silver wire" changes are noted at the superior disk margin and irregular narrowing of the artery is noted on the left superior side of the figure.

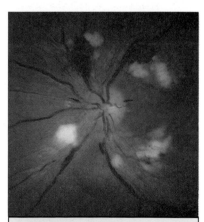

Fig. 245 Stage III malignant hypertension with cotton-wool spots, flame-shaped hemorrhages, and arteriolar narrowing.

Retinal hemorrhages

Retinal vein occlusions cause a painless decrease in vision with hemorrhages extending to the peripheral retina. Acutely, there are flame-shaped hemorrhages (see Fig. 247, p. 87) and blot hemorrhages (see Fig. 248, p. 87). The flame hemorrhages clear as collaterals develop on the disk in several months. Dot hemorrhages (see Fig. 248, p. 87) may last for years. Cottonwool spots and a poorly reactive pupil usually indicate an ischemic retina due to a total occlusion. Ischemia is confirmed with fluorescein angiography. In this case, the visual prognosis is poor. Laser photocoagulation may limit edema of the macula or cause regression of rubeosis iridis, which occurs in 30% of cases.

Retinal blood vessels appear white when inflamed. Arteritis occurs in sarcoidosis (Fig. 244), cytomegalovirus retinitis, and lupus erythematosis. Phlebitis occurs in Eales' disease, an inflammatory condition in young boys. Damaged vessels from choroiditis and vein and artery occlusions could develop a white fibrous sheathing (see Fig. 253, p. 88), or appear thread-like since there is no circulation.

Hypertensive retinopathy

Scheie classification		
I	Thinning of retinal arterioles relative to veins	Stages I and II are similar to arteriosclerosis of aging
II	Obvious arteriolar narrowing with focal areas of attenuation (Fig. 243)	
III	Stage II, plus cotton-wool spots, exudates, and hemorrhages (Fig. 245)	Stages III and IV are medical emergencies referred to as malignant hypertension. Ninety percent die in 1 year if not treated
IV	Stage III plus swollen optic disk resembling papilledema	

Depths of retinal hemorrhages

(Figs 246—250)

Preretinal hemorrhages (Fig. 246)

Preretinal hemorrhages occur between the vitreous and retina and may layer out to a boat shape. They are caused by proliferative diabetic retinopathy with breakthrough into vitreous. Trauma and vitreous detachments are also common causes.

Superficial flame-shaped hemorrhages (Fig. 247)

These occur in the nerve fiber layer radiating from the optic disk. They are caused by central retinal vein occlusion. They are also common in papilledema, diabetes, hypertension, and optic neuritis (see Fig. 60, p. 24).

Deep retinal hemorrhages (Fig. 248)

Dot and blot hemorrhages occur most often in diabetes, papilledema, and venostasis conditions such as 1-year-old retinal vein occlusion (Fig. 248).

Subretinal hemorrhages (Fig. 249)

In disciform macular degeneration these are darker red under the retinal pigment epithelium (RPE) than in the sensory retina. Retinal vessels overlie deep hemorrhages.

Retinal artery occlusion

Retinal artery occlusion (Fig. 251) causes sudden loss of vision. Carotid artery plaques (see Fig. 77, p. 34) or heart disease such as arrhythmias, endocarditis, or valve disease may liberate fine platelets or larger cholesterol emboli (Hollenhorst plaque), which lodge in arterial bifurcations. Sludging of blood flow gives a box-car appearance (Fig. 252). The resulting ischemic retina becomes edematous giving the macula a cherry-red appearance. Irreparable loss of vision occurs within 1 hour. Eventually optic atrophy results

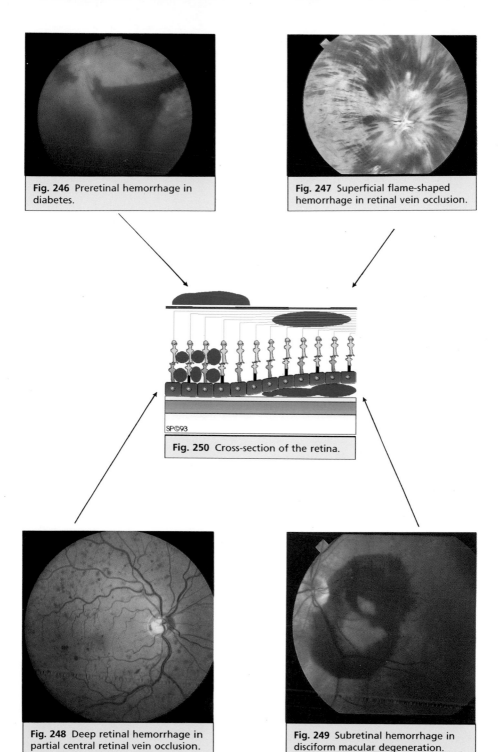

Fig. 246 Preretinal hemorrhage in diabetes.

Fig. 247 Superficial flame-shaped hemorrhage in retinal vein occlusion.

Fig. 250 Cross-section of the retina.

Fig. 248 Deep retinal hemorrhage in partial central retinal vein occlusion.

Fig. 249 Subretinal hemorrhage in disciform macular degeneration.

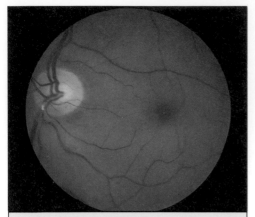

Fig. 251 Retinal artery occlusion with Hollenhorst plaque on disk with cherry-red macula. See Fig. 233, p. 80.

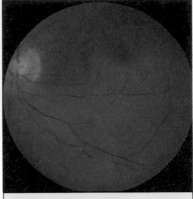

Fig. 252 Box-car sludging in arteries.

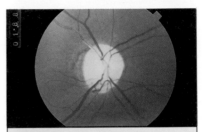

Fig. 253 Late-stage retinal artery occlusion with optic atrophy and arteries that are thread-like and sheathed.

(Fig. 253). Rx: 95% O_2/5% CO_2 inhalation to dilate the artery and intravenous Diamox to lower pressure. Massage the eye to get embolus to move on. Call ophthalmologist immediately to tap anterior chamber, which lowers eye pressure.

Diabetic retinopathy

There are three progressive stages of diabetic retinopathy.

1 Nonproliferative or background retinopathy presents initially with microaneurysms (Fig. 254). Aneurysms leak (Fig. 255) and cause edema and proteinaceous exudate at the macula, which is the most common reason for loss of vision in diabetes. Later, dot hemorrhages appear. Laser photocoagulation may reduce leakage that threatens the macula.

2 Preproliferative retinopathy (Fig. 256) is due to widespread capillary closure (Fig. 257) causing retinal ischemia as indicated by cotton-wool spots, venous beading, and larger blot hemorrhages.

3 Proliferative diabetic retinopathy begins with fine tufts of capillaries on or around the disk (Fig. 258). They may bleed into the vitreous and cause fibrotic membranes (Fig. 259) that contract and cause retinal detachments. Pan-retinal photocoagulation destroys part of

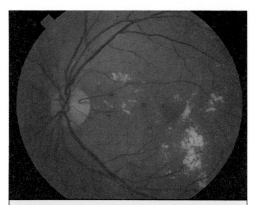

Fig. 254 Stage 1. Background retinopathy with microaneurysms and exudates.

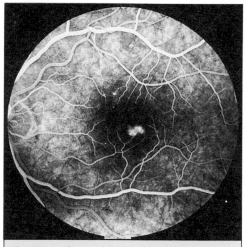

Fig. 255 Leakage of fluorescein from microaneurysms. Normal retinal vessels do not leak.

the ischemic retina thus reducing some of the stimulus that causes neovascularization. This third stage often occurs late in the course of diabetes and is associated with other serious systemic vascular diseases and an associated 56% 5-year survival.

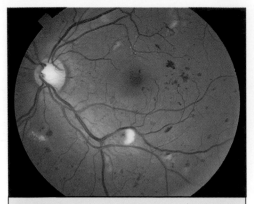

Fig. 256 Stage 2. Preproliferative retinopathy with cotton-wool spot.

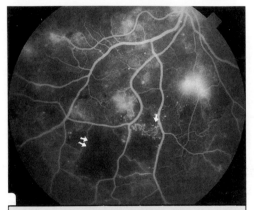

Fig. 257 Fluorescein angiogram showing neovascularization adjacent to dark area of capillary nonperfusion.

Macular degeneration

Age-related macular degeneration is the leading cause of blindness in elderly persons. Twenty-five percent of 70-year-old persons have signs of the condition and this number increases to 50% by age 90. In a normal retina (Fig. 260), the RPE has tight junctions protecting the sensory retina from leakage of more permeable choroidal capillaries. The RPE also metabolically supports the rods and cones and creates an adhesive force with the overlying neurosensory retina, which prevents retinal detachments.

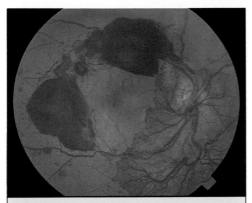

Fig. 258 Stage 3a. Proliferative retinopathy with neovascularization and preretinal hemorrhages.

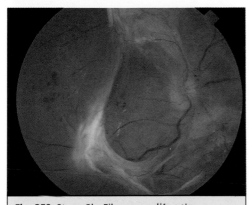

Fig. 259 Stage 3b. Fibrous proliferation.

In macular degeneration, Bruch's membrane degenerates by fragmenting in some areas and thickening with hyaline (drusen) in other areas (Figs 228 and 261). The RPE on top of the drusen degenerates. The overlying sensory retina dependent on the RPE thins out resulting in atrophic (nonexudative) macular degeneration (Figs 261 and 262). This accounts for 70% of all cases of macular degeneration. If enough retina disappears, the choroidal vasculature is easily visualized.

Ten percent of macular degeneration is due to the disciform (exudative) type (Figs 263–266). This occurs when blood vessels from the choroid penetrate the damaged Bruch's membrane (subretinal neovascularitization). These

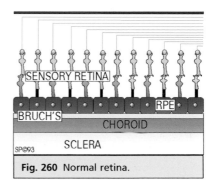

Fig. 260 Normal retina.

vessels may bleed causing a hemorrhagic detachment of the RPE, which appears dark red. When it breaks into the sensory retina, it appears bright red (Fig. 266). Eventually, the blood fibroses and forms a white scar. A fluorescein angiogram may reveal the subretinal vessels before they bleed (Fig. 264).

If the neovascular membrane is more than 200 μm from the fovea it can be safely destroyed with argon laser photocoagulation. Both atrophic and disciform degeneration have an onset after age 50. Early signs of both are drusen, pigment mottling at the macular, loss of foveal reflexes, decreased central vision, and waviness of lines on Amsler grid testing. Both types might benefit from taking antioxidant vitamins A, E, and C with zinc. Ultraviolet light damages the macula and filters are of value.

The remaining 20% of macular degenerations are due to juvenile inherited types, chorioretinitis, infection, and staring at the sun. Reassure patients that they never go totally blind, but only lose central vision often resulting in 20/400 vision.

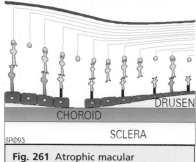

Fig. 261 Atrophic macular degeneration.

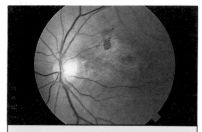

Fig. 262 Atrophic macular degeneration.

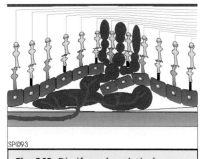

Fig. 263 Disciform (exudative) macular degeneration.

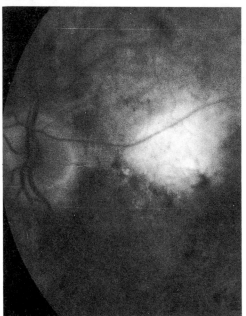

Fig. 264 Fluorescein angiogram of subretinal neovascular membrane.

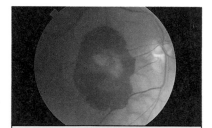

Fig. 265 Hemorrhagic stage of disciform macular degeneration.

Common retinal diseases

Central serous retinopathy

This is a macular disease in which a defect in the RPE allows choroidal fluid to leak into the sensory retina (Figs 267–269). It usually affects males ages 25–40 and may be triggered by stress. Symptoms are decreased and distorted vision. Wavy lines are demonstrated with an Amsler grid. Ophthalmoscopically, there is a clear oval elevation of retina. Eighty to ninety percent clear within a few months. Laser photocoagulation may be used if leakage continues for 6 months.

Retinal detachments

These are separations of the neurosensory retina from the RPE (Fig. 270). They often begin with degeneration in the peripheral retina, such as myopic thinning or lattice degeneration. Lattice degeneration is seen with an indirect ophthalmoscope in 8% of eyes as a white meshwork of lines with black pigment near the ora serrata (Fig. 271). Holes may develop in these areas spontaneously or from trauma, cataract surgery, vitreous traction, or contraction of diabetic retinal membranes. Fluid then enters the holes and detaches the retina (Fig. 272). Not all holes cause problems. Small, round, asymptomatic holes may often be left untreated. Large horseshoe tears with vitreous traction and recent symptoms must be sealed. Symptoms include loss of vision,

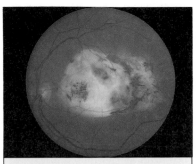

Fig. 266 Late-stage disciform scar. Courtesy of Leo Masciulli.

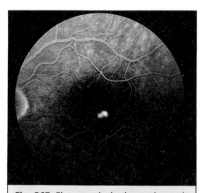

Fig. 267 Fluorescein leakage through the RPE in central serous retinopathy.

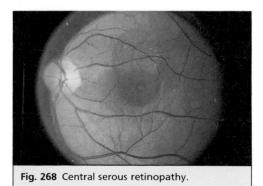

Fig. 268 Central serous retinopathy.

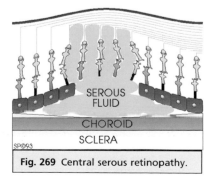

SEROUS FLUID

CHOROID

SCLERA

SP©93

Fig. 269 Central serous retinopathy.

described as a "curtain," with flashes and floaters. Ophthalmoscopically, an elevated gray membrane is seen unless a vitreous hemorrhage obscures it. At surgery (Fig. 273), the subretinal fluid is drained through a scleral hole. The retinal hole and surrounding retina is then scarred to underlying choroid using laser, cryopexy, or diathermy. A scleral buckle is placed, which pushes the sclera against the retina.

Distortion of central vision with an irregular reflex and associated vitreous traction could indicate the onset of a macular hole. Macular holes (Fig. 274) do not usually lead to detachments, but if they are full thickness, central vision could drop to 20/400. A vitrectomy could prevent progression to a full-thickness hole.

Albinism

Albinism has many forms and refers to inherited hypopigmentation. Common findings in all types involving the eye are photophobia, hypopigmentation of the retina (Fig. 275), and transillumination of the iris with a penlight at the limbus (Fig. 276). Additional findings may include nystagmus, a hypoplastic macula with absence of a foveal reflex, reduced vision, refractive errors, decreased pigmentation of hair and skin, and decreased immunity (Fig. 277).

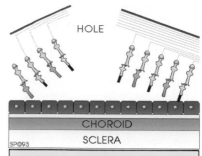
Fig. 270 Retinal hole with detachment of sensory retina.

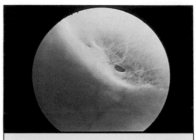
Fig. 271 Lattice degeneration with round hole. Courtesy of Leo Bores.

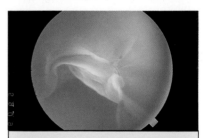
Fig. 272 Retinal detachment with large hole.

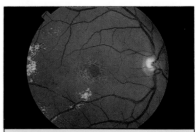
Fig. 274 Macular hole in diabetic with exudates.

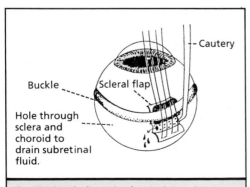
Fig. 273 Surgical repair of retinal detachment.

Retinitis pigmentosa (Fig. 278)

This is a slowly progressive hereditary degeneration. Since it begins in the retinal periphery, the first loss is peripheral and night vision (Fig. 279), often sparing central visual acuity for many years. The retina has pigmentary changes resembling bone corpuscles. Diagnosis is confirmed with an electroretinogram.

A study released in May 1993 showed that 15 000 IU of vitamin A given daily to 601 patients slowed retinal damage as shown by electroretinogram findings. There is as yet no correlation with improvement in visual loss.

Retinoblastoma (Figs 280 and 281)

This is a malignant tumor of the retina often appearing by 2 years of age. Most occur from a genetic mutation that survivors may transmit as a mendelian dominant. The retina has one or more white elevated retinal masses, which are bilateral 30% of the time. Removal of the eye is indicated for unilateral cases. When both eyes are involved, the worst eye may be enucleated and the other treated with chemo-, radio-, laser-, or cryotherapy.

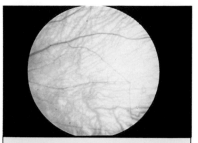

Fig. 275 Albinotic fundus.

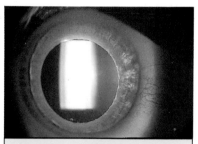

Fig. 276 Transilluminated iris.

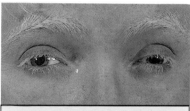

Fig. 277 Albinotic hair and skin.

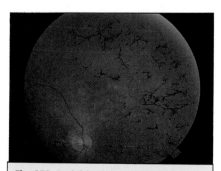

Fig. 278 Retinitis pigmentosa.

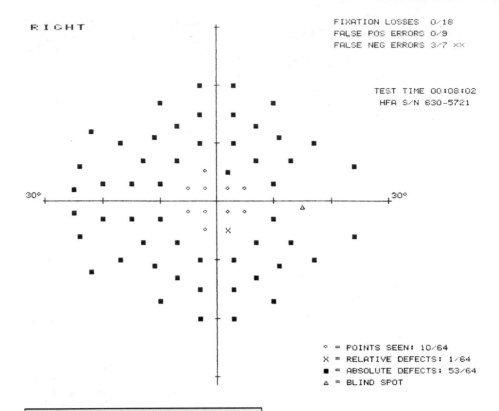

FIXATION LOSSES 0/18
FALSE POS ERRORS 0/9
FALSE NEG ERRORS 3/7 ××

TEST TIME 00:08:02
HFA S/N 830-5721

30°　　　　　　　　　　　　　　　　　　　　　30°

○ = POINTS SEEN: 10/64
× = RELATIVE DEFECTS: 1/64
■ = ABSOLUTE DEFECTS: 53/64
△ = BLIND SPOT

Fig. 279 Constricted visual field in late-stage retinitis pigmentosa. Dark squares indicate absence of vision.

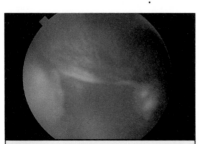

Fig. 280 Retinoblastoma. Courtesy of David Taylor.

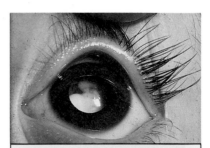

Fig. 281 Leukocoria (white pupil) due to retinoblastoma.

Retinopathy of prematurity

This condition is bilateral in premature infants less than 3 lb in weight, and usually in those given oxygen. Normal vascularization of the retina progresses peripherally and is not normally completed until 1 month after birth. Oxygen given to newborns stops this normal vascularization process. When the oxygen is discontinued the avascular peripheral retina stimulates new vessel growth (Fig. 283). These new vessels, however, are now abnormal and may bleed resulting in vitreous hemorrhage with fibrous proliferation. It could drag the retina (Fig. 284), sometimes causing a retinal detachment. The ideal therapy is reduction in the number of premature births and careful monitoring of oxygen in the nursery. An ophthalmologist should check the peripheral retina when the baby leaves the nursery and again at 3 months. Transscleral cryotherapy may be used to scar the avascular retina in severe cases.

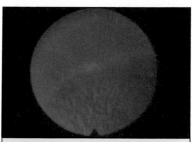

Fig. 283 Retinopathy of prematurity: demarcation line between normal and avascular retina. Anteriorly to this line neovascular tufts can be seen. Courtesy of David Taylor.

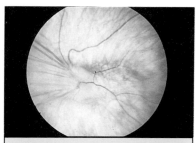

Fig. 284 Late-stage of retinopathy of prematurity with disk and retinal vessels dragged peripherally on left side.

Appendix

Characteristics of three causes of an inflamed eye			
	Iritis	*Conjunctivitis*	*Acute glaucoma*
Symptom	Pain, photophobia	Gritty, itching	Severe pain
Discharge	Tearing	Pus, mucous,	Tearing
Pupil	Miotic	Normal	Mid-dilated
Injection	Limbal	Diffuse	Diffuse and limbal
Cornea	Keratitic precipitates	Clear	Steamy cornea
Pressure	Usually low	Normal	Elevated
Anterior chamber	Flare and cells	Normal	Shallow